THE MENOPAUSE

An Essential Guide by Nicci Talbot

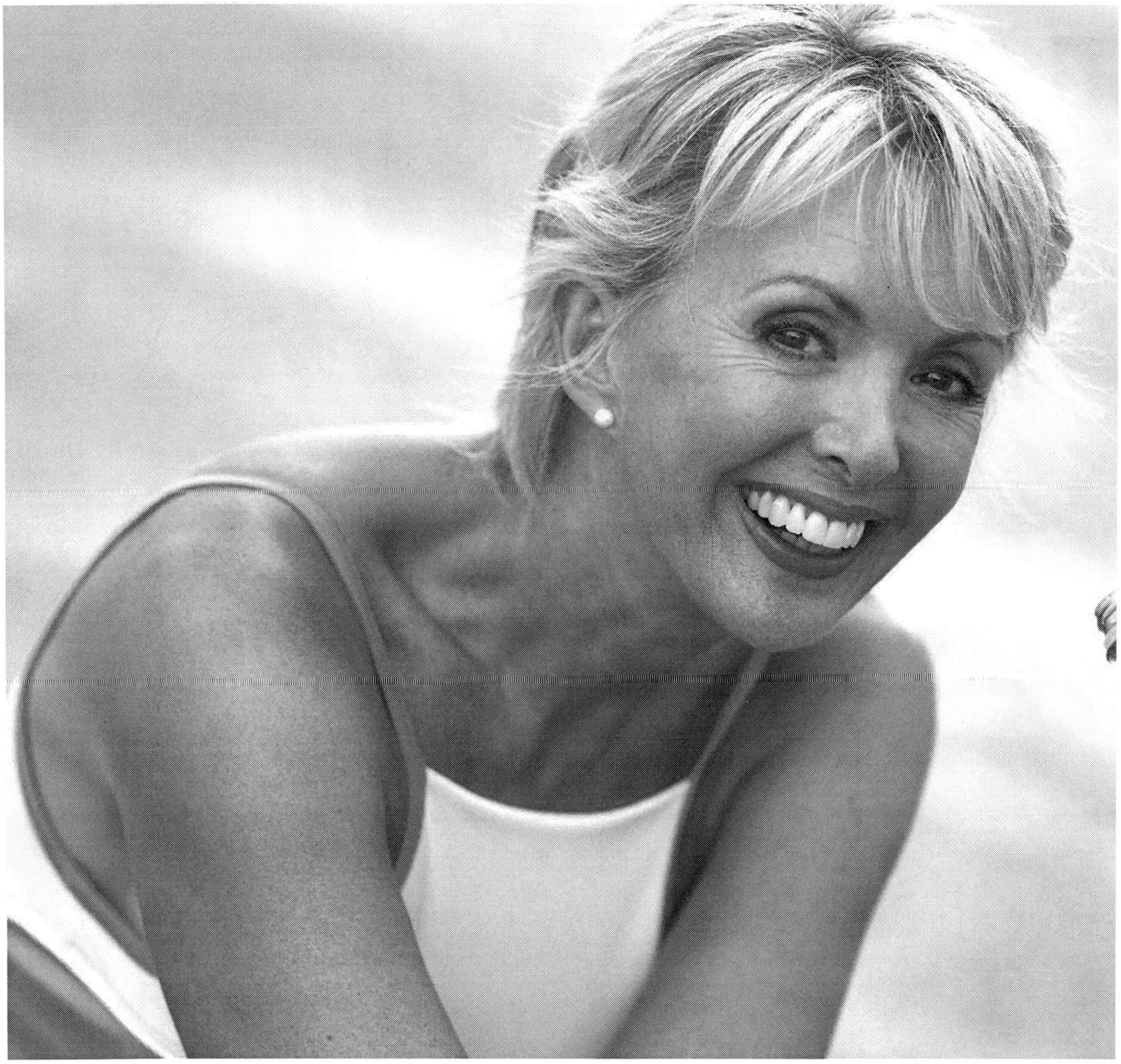

First published in Great Britain in 2009 by
Need2Know
Remus House
Coltsfoot Drive
Peterborough
PE2 9JX
Telephone 01733 898103
Fax 01733 313524
www.need2knowbooks.co.uk

Large Print Edition 2011 (based on 2009 version).

Need2Know is an imprint of Bonacia Ltd.

SB ISBN 978-1-86144-167-6
Cover photograph: Jupiter Images
Author photograph: John Malloch-Caldwell

Contents

Introduction

'Prolonged use of HRT increases breast cancer risks, researchers warn.'

'HRT linked to ovarian cancer risk.'

'HRT pills may double risk of blood clot but patches deemed "safe".'

If you've been diagnosed as menopausal and offered hormone replacement therapy (HRT) by your GP, news reports like these might make you feel a bit anxious. HRT is a controversial treatment that doesn't suit everyone, yet it seems to be commonly prescribed for menopausal women. There is a lot of misinformation and much of the media coverage has focused on the negative effects of long term trials. So who are we to believe? What does it do and how safe is it? There are over 50 different types on the market, so how do you know which is best for you? And if you've already decided that you prefer a more holistic approach, what are your options?

The menopause can be a stressful time – it has become medicalised to a degree despite being a natural event in every woman's life. You will have lots of questions about what is happening to your body and you'll want to know what your options are and how to safeguard your health in the long term. However, it can be difficult to uncover the facts and express your feelings in a 10 minute appointment with your GP. That's where this book can help. It presents key information that you need to know about the menopause and will help you decide on the best course of action. It explains what the menopause is, the different stages, what to expect and how to deal with common symptoms on a day-to-day basis.

70% of women experience physical, sexual and psychological symptoms during the perimenopause (the period leading up the menopause). These can include hot flushes, irregular periods and vaginal changes, aching joints, night sweats, anxiety and a lack of concentration. This can be distressing when you're used to a highly efficient body and mind that works to order! It can feel like you're not in control of your body anymore and, as this stage can last for several years, you'll probably wonder if you'll ever feel like your old self again. Many women don't seek medical help for these symptoms – they put them down to 'the change' and soldier on as normal. However, there's no reason why you should put up with anything that disrupts your quality of life. You can alleviate your symptoms naturally and this guide explains how.

More women are choosing to use complementary therapies to help treat menopausal symptoms instead of (or in addition to) medical treatments like HRT. There are many different types of complementary therapy and this book will look at the most useful ones for the menopause. There are also chapters on diet and nutrition, sex, exercise and other changes you can make to ease your symptoms and protect your health against common conditions in later life such as osteoporosis and heart disease.

There are many myths and preconceptions about the menopause which aren't challenged because women don't really talk about how they are feeling or what they are going through. It's something that is joked about and swept under the carpet rather than celebrated as a rite of passage in every woman's life. In many cultures menopausal women are considered wise, with life lessons to share. This is how it should be, yet somehow along the way we've lost a bit of respect for our bodies, elevating youth and beauty over life experience.

The menopause is an individual experience, affecting every woman differently. It needs to be treated holistically. Some women will sail through it with hardly any symptoms, for others it will have an impact on their lives. However, it shouldn't be a negative experience. This is a new stage in your life, a period of transition and an opportunity to assess where you are now and to reflect on what you've achieved so far and what you want for your future. This guide will help you to do just that.

Disclaimer

This guide is for general information about the menopause only. This book is not intended to replace professional medical advice. Anyone with serious concerns about their health or menopause symptoms should contact their GP or healthcare professional immediately.

Acknowledgements

With thanks to the following for advice and help:
Julie G Silver, Optimum Health Consultancy
Georgia Foster, Hypnotherapy
Carole Ann Rice, Life Coaching
Val Sampson, Relationship Counselling
Fiona Kirk, Nutritionalist
Lucy Wyndham-Read, Fitness Training
Miranda Gray, Optimised Woman
Sue & Hilly at Shakti Tantra
Paul & Sam at Jo Divine
Dr John Moran at the Holistic Medical Clinic
Victoria Health Pharmacy
All the lovely ladies who took the time to respond to my menopause questionnaire.

All About the Menopause (1)

What is the menopause?

The menopause is the transition from reproductive to non-reproductive life. It is referred to as the 'change of life' or 'climacteric'.

As we age, our ovaries gradually start to wind down and stop producing as much oestrogen and progesterone, which has an impact on how our body and brain function. Ovulation becomes less frequent and eventually you have your final period. With a natural menopause, this process takes years. The first sign is usually erratic periods which can be heavier than normal. You may have two in one month and then nothing for ages. The average age for menopause in the UK is 51. However, it can occur between 45 and 55 years of age – each woman is different and when it happens is down to genetics, lifestyle factors and medical history.

Most of the discussion about the menopause and its effects centres on the beginning stage, known as the perimenopause, when your ovaries are still functioning but gradually start to slow down. This is when the classic symptoms of hot flushes, night sweats and erratic periods arise, and when you might start to think about ways of replacing the declining hormones. While your body readjusts to lower levels of oestrogen, these symptoms can range in severity – from bothersome to seriously uncomfortable.

During the perimenopause your body continues to produce oestrogen in the adrenal glands and ovaries but in smaller amounts. You may ovulate one month and not the next, even though you are still having regular periods. This can be a confusing time of emotional highs and lows as your body tries to compensate for the decline of oestrogen. As journalist Gail Sheehy explains in her book The Silent Passage, it can be quite a shock to realise you are perimenopausal.

The menopause itself is a retrospective event, defined as occurring when it's been a year since your last period. At this point you have ceased ovulation and you can no longer get pregnant, and you might have mixed emotions about this. On the one hand, you may feel sad that you can no longer bear children and on the other, relieved of the burden of monthly periods and contraceptive routines. Many women have commented that it is quite a nice feeling to be free of periods and reproductive demands.

The menopause is a metamorphosis and a positive event. However, there is still quite a lot of negativity, misinformation and prejudice about this stage in a woman's life which can make it an anxious time. This book will dispel some of those myths and give you an insight into what is happening to your body and how you can best manage it, according to your preferences. No two women will experience the same menopause – women online (Good Housekeeping forum – www.allaboutyou.com) have used a colour scale from mild pink to raging scarlet to describe the severity of their symptoms!

Stages of menopause

The menopause is broken down into the following stages:

- Premenopause – refers to a woman's reproductive life from first menstruation to menopause.
- Perimenopause – typically starting in your mid forties, this is a period of flux as the ovaries gradually start to wind down and produce fewer hormones. This stage can last anything from two to six years with an average of 3.8 years according to a survey by the World Health Organisation. Your periods usually become erratic and heavier than normal. You may still be ovulating but less oestrogen is produced. Your ovaries are no longer responding to messages from the brain. They start to slow down production of oestrogen and progesterone, meaning that fewer eggs are being produced. Low levels of hormones mean the womb lining isn't being stimulated enough for your period to start. This chemical activity in the brain triggers hot flushes and

night sweats. You may also notice other changes such as vaginal dryness, aching joints and mood swings. If your symptoms are affecting your quality of life, talk to your GP and complementary health practitioner about options for treatment. Prolonged heavy bleeding could be a sign of further health issues such as fibroids or endometriosis and needs to be checked out as soon as possible.

- Menopause – this is a retrospective event because it doesn't actually happen until it's been one full year since your last period. You may go four months without a period and then have an unexpected one. Nature has a strange sense of humour at times! This is why experts recommend maintaining contraception for a year after your final period if you are over 50. Pregnancy is unlikely at this stage but has been known to happen.
- Postmenopause – this is the rest of your life once it's been a year since your last period. Nowadays, we can expect to live for around 30 years after the menopause, so planning for long-term health and wellbeing is paramount.

Although the menopause is divided into distinct stages, 'menopause' is the general term to encompass all of the above.

A brief history

The word 'menopause' comes from the Greek words 'menos' and 'pausis', meaning to come to an end. In the 1800s, French physician De Gardanne mentioned the term 'la menopause'. Around this time 'bad humours' in the body were thought to cause illness and were eradicated by unpleasant means such as leeching. The discovery of the endocrine system and the role hormones play in menopausal symptoms and our health came later. Louise Foxcroft's book Hot Flushes, Cold Science: A History of Modern Menopause provides an insight into how the menopause was perceived and how things have changed.

During the 19th century women were considered hysterical (womb being the word for hysteria) during the climacteric. It was thought that the ovaries were the root of this and when they stopped functioning women lost the plot, becoming sexual deviants or mad. So, the only way to cure a woman of her 'madness' was to remove her ovaries – an unpleasant operation prior to anaesthetic. Doctors also had the onerous task of relieving women of their 'hysteria' (libido) by masturbating them to orgasm with old-style vibrators, as Rachel P Maines explains in her book The Technology of Orgasm. Thankfully, things have advanced since then and we now know that the symptoms of menopause are caused by hormone deficiency, and we have more civilised ways of treating this via hormone replacement therapy.

An alternative view in ancient times, explains psychotherapist and life coach Dr Daphne Stevens, who runs holistic menopause workshops for women, was that the blood normally expelled during your period was retained in the womb after the menopause to nourish a woman's growing wisdom that developed with age. Hence the delightful term 'wise blood'. This view is upheld today in several indigenous cultures around the world where elder tribeswomen are respected within their communities, allowed to participate and give wise counsel once they reach the menopause. They are regarded as healers and wise women, and take on the role of advising and helping younger girls move into womanhood.

Think of the menopause as a pause rather than cessation. You are coming up for air after years of working hard, childbearing and building and maintaining relationships. It's time to reassess the next stage – 'me time' – and to put some new plans into action for the future.

Premature menopause

This is when a woman experiences menopause before she reaches the age of 40. Around one in 100 women will experience this according to the support charity The Daisy Network. The causes can be surgical as result of a hysterectomy or oophorectomy (removal of the ovaries), or after radiotherapy or chemotherapy to treat cancer. This can damage the ovaries and affect their production of oestrogen. Pelvic surgery is another cause as it exposes the ovaries to chemicals, and partial hysterectomy (with ovaries intact) can also bring on the menopause a little earlier.

Lifestyle factors that influence early menopause include smoking (roughly two years earlier) because it affects ovarian function. Hereditary factors and overexposure to chemicals at work also have a part to play.

The Wallace-Kelsey test

This test was designed by Scottish scientists Dr Thomas Kelsey and Dr Hamish Wallace to help predict the menopause. They hypothesised that it is possible to predict when the menopause is likely to happen within two to three years by measuring the size of a woman's ovaries and how many eggs she has left. Research is currently ongoing into how accurate this is. It's possible to have the test done privately – more information can be found in the help list.

Diagnostic testing

If you're starting to experience symptoms of perimenopause, your first port of call is your GP. Request a female doctor if you prefer or contact your local Well Woman Clinic which will have in-depth information and testing available (clinics can be found in your doctor's surgery or local hospital. They offer advice on gynaecological problems, contraception, smear testing, breast checks, HRT and the menopause). Tests will be carried out to measure your hormone levels: follicle stimulating hormone (FSH) and luteinising hormone (LH). Repeated high levels of FSH in the blood indicate that the menopause is approaching.

Your womb and ovaries may also be checked for fibroids or cysts. It's also important to check your thyroid levels for diabetes and your bone density if you have a family history of osteoporosis.

What your GP will need to know

If you decide that it is time to visit your GP, it is worth preparing a list of questions and thoughts based on your medical history and observations so far. They will need to know:

- What form of contraception you are using.
- How your periods are – regular, infrequent, heavy or scant.
- Personal and family medical history.
- What supplements, vitamins or complementary therapies you are using.
- How you feel about the menopause and taking HRT. Do you prefer a holistic approach to the menopause?
- What method of HRT administration you would prefer.

Checklist

- Think about what kind of approach you want to take – holistic or HRT/drugs?
- Keep a diary, charting any observations or symptoms you notice and any triggers for them.
- What do you want from the next stage of your life? Are you taking on new work which requires stamina and energy or are you planning to take things more slowly and develop your own interests?
- Do you have the contact details for your local Well Woman Clinic?
- Make a list of questions for your GP.

Summing Up

The menopause is a natural transition from reproductive to non-reproductive life. The average age for this is 51. As we age, our ovaries begin to wind down and produce less oestrogen. We ovulate less frequently and eventually have our final period. The menopause itself is a retrospective event, defined as having occurred when it has been a year since your last period.

The menopause is separated into three different stages: premenopause, perimenopause and postmenopause. Premenopause is from puberty (your first period) until your final period. Perimenopause typically starts in the mid-40s and lasts, on average, 3.8 years. The postmenopausal years are those following your final period.

Different tests are available to determine when the menopause is likely to occur. The Wallace-Kelsey test is based on the size of a woman's ovaries and how many eggs she has left. You can also have tests done to measure your hormone levels, particularly FSH as high levels indicate that the menopause is approaching. Ask your GP for more details.

The Reproductive Cycle (2)

Before we look at symptoms and solutions, we need an understanding of the reproductive cycle and the hormones involved.

The average menstrual cycle is 28 days. Here's how the cycle works during your reproductive years.

The follicular phase (day 1-14)

Oestrogen and progesterone levels are low at the start of the cycle. This makes the womb shed its lining and starts your period. Oestrogen levels gradually rise, reaching a peak mid-cycle (around day 14) when you ovulate. You will notice you feel sunnier and more energetic while this process is happening as high levels of oestrogen promote good mood and wellbeing. Your libido also rises, peaking around ovulation as your body tries its best to get you pregnant.

This process is controlled by hormones – FSH (follicle stimulating hormone) and LH (luteinising hormone). These are controlled by the pituitary gland in the brain. They tell the ovaries to produce oestrogen and progesterone at the right time and stimulate the development of between 3-30 follicles and the release of an egg from one of these into the fallopian tubes.

The ovulatory phase (6-32 hours)

There is a surge in LH and ovulation takes place. One of the follicles releases an egg from one ovary which you can sometimes feel as a dull ache on your left or right side of the lower stomach/pelvic area. The egg has 12 hours to be fertilised for pregnancy to occur.

The luteal phase (days 15-28)

This is the second half of your cycle, after ovulation has taken place. Oestrogen levels begin to decline and progesterone is dominant to help prepare the womb for possible pregnancy. If the egg isn't fertilised, the follicle dies and becomes an empty shell known as the corpus luteum. This is shed by the endometrium and you get your period. Your brain releases more FSH to stimulate the process to start all over again. High amounts of progesterone during the luteal phase give rise to typical symptoms of PMS – breast tenderness, bloating, mood swings and sugary cravings.

The optimized woman

For an insight into how the menstrual cycle affects your moods, cognitive thinking and energy levels, read Miranda Gray's book The Optimized Woman. As Gray explains, certain times of the month are more productive than others for setting goals and tackling different tasks. It helps to work with your body rather than against it.

The menstrual cycle at menopause

This cycle runs pretty smoothly throughout your reproductive life. However, things begin to change as you reach the perimenopause because hormone levels start to decline and your ovaries produce fewer eggs. The follicular phase gets shorter, ovulation may not occur every month and less progesterone is being made. Your body is producing unopposed oestrogen which makes the endometrium lining grow thicker. The result being erratic, heavy periods. Your brain tries to correct this imbalance by pumping out greater levels of FSH and LH to stimulate the ovaries. Consequently, all of this hormonal activity can make you feel very irritable, tired and out of sorts.

As you near the menopause, your hormone levels become so low that menstruation isn't possible. Your body continues to produce oestrogen from the adrenal glands but in a much weaker form.

Hormones

The word hormone comes from the Greek word 'hormon' which means to stir things up. Hormones don't have a direct job – they are chemical messengers which means they pave the way for things to happen in the body; they enable our bodies and brains to function at their prime. Most of the time we don't even think about what they do because they do their job so well. It's only when things start to change (at puberty and during the perimenopause) that we realise how powerful they are and what an impact they have on our health.

Your hormones

The ovaries produce three hormones: oestrogen, progesterone and testosterone. These have a yin and yang principle – they balance each other out and work together to help your body function. They have a huge impact on your sexual functioning and sense of wellbeing. Below is a brief outline of what they do.

Oestrogen

Oestrogen is produced in the ovaries and plays a big role in puberty, genital and breast development. We have receptor sites for oestrogen all over our bodies. At puberty it gives us our womanly shape, hip to waist ratio and breasts as an indicator of fertility. However, it also has a protective effect and keeps the heart and brain healthy. It keeps the vaginal lining smooth and moist, enables lubrication and takes care of the urinary tract. It also makes the vagina receptive to sperm by changing the texture of cervical mucus so that it is thinner, enabling sperm to pass through to the egg. On an exterior level, it keeps our skin and hair thick and shiny. It is a very powerful hormone.

There are three types of oestrogen:

- Oestrodial – this is the strongest form which powers the menstrual cycle and reproduction.

- Oestrone – this is a weaker form that is present postmenopause. It is made in the ovaries prior to the menopause and by fat cells after the menopause. Women who have more body fat may reach the menopause later because oestrone is still being produced in low amounts.
- Oestriol – this is present during pregnancy.

Collectively, the three types are referred to as oestrogen.

Progesterone

Progesterone is also produced in the ovaries after ovulation has taken place. Its main job is preparing the endometrium for pregnancy and helping to support the pregnancy until the foetus can produce its own hormones. In the luteal phase of your cycle it has a huge effect on your moods, giving rise to typical PMS symptoms such as tender breasts, food cravings, bloating and low mood.

Follicle stimulating hormone (FSH)

This is produced in the pituitary gland and starts the ovulation process by directing the ovaries to start producing follicles.

Luteinising hormone (LH)

This is produced in the pituitary gland and tells the developed follicle to release an egg for the ovulation phase of the cycle.

Testosterone

This is produced in the ovaries in smaller amounts. During the perimenopause, levels rise slightly to compensate for the drop in oestrogen production. This can give you a surge in libido and other noticeable side effects such as hair growth in unwanted places. It has various functions, including stimulating hair production, regulating libido and promoting bone and muscle growth. It also contributes to your changing body shape from pear to apple-shaped around the waist.

Checklist

- Do you know how long your menstrual cycle is?
- Take a note of the different stages and the effects they have on your mood. See Miranda Gray's book The Optimized Woman for further details.
- Chart your cycle for a month and observe when you feel most sociable, creative and have good levels of concentration and motivation. Make a plan to work with this cycle next time you have your period.

Summing Up

The average menstrual cycle is 28 days long. It consists of the follicular phase (day one of your period to day 14). Your hormone levels gradually rise, peaking at ovulation (around day 14 of your cycle). This puts you in a good mood and promotes high energy levels. The ovulatory phase lasts between 6-32 hours and pregnancy is possible during this time. The luteal phase is the second half of your cycle post-ovulation, when oestrogen levels decline and progesterone levels rise to prepare your body for a period or pregnancy. Higher levels of progesterone contribute to typical PMS symptoms of breast tenderness, bloating and mood swings.

During the perimenopause this cycle changes due to falling oestrogen levels and the fact that you may not ovulate every month. The follicular phase gets shorter and less progesterone is made. Your brain tries to compensate by pumping out extra hormones which makes you feel out of sorts.

Hormones are chemical messengers that pave the way for things to happen in the body. The key sex hormones are oestrogen, progesterone and testosterone. These pave the way for puberty, menstruation and pregnancy and also help maintain libido, healthy bones and a sense of wellbeing.

Symptoms and Solutions (3)

Common physical symptoms

Some women go through the menopause with minimal symptoms. However, 80% of women will experience physical, sexual and emotional symptoms and will find it hard to cope. You might be having mild hot flushes that are bothersome but haven't found the time to see your GP about it. For others, the flushes and heavy periods will be debilitating, affecting daily life. It's best to seek advice early on even if you're not sure whether you are actually perimenopausal. Heavy periods always need to be investigated to rule out any other health concerns.

Kathryn Colas, founder of the menopause support website Simply Hormones, urges women to make changes as early as possible: 'It was a negative time in my life to begin with but now I have found my own path to wellness again. I urge women to approach menopausal symptoms sooner rather than later. The sooner, the better, as I believe a natural pathway can be successful, but you must be committed to making changes to your lifestyle'.

Menopausal symptoms such as anxiety, hot flushes and mood swings will be exacerbated by stress, so it's important to take a look at your lifestyle. Try to re-evaluate what is important and what you can let go – relationships included. Evie Abston, a blogger for Good Vibrations sex store, suggests that hot flushes are your body's way of bringing up issues that need to be dealt with. It helps to see them as empowering and a form of detox. Perimenopause can be a tricky time – you may have teenage children leaving home, elderly parents to take care of and a partner with his/her own issues to deal with, all of which can have a bearing on your health and wellbeing.

This chapter outlines some of the most common menopausal symptoms and their causes. It's a rather long list, but don't panic – the chances of you experiencing all of them are very slim! Start making changes to your lifestyle now, tackling any problems as they arise, and you will find it easier to cope. Eat well, exercise and stay motivated and busy. Maintain your social networks and talk to other women about what you're experiencing. The online health and wellbeing magazine forums such as Good Housekeeping, Prima and Woman and Home are a great place to read about other women's experiences. You will see that you are not alone!

You may also find it helpful at this stage to keep a diary of symptoms to show your GP and complementary health practitioner. It's easy to forget when things are happening and what treatments you have tried unless you make a note of it.

Menstrual changes

Irregular bleeding and heavy periods

As explained in chapter 2, during the perimenopause your ovaries are producing less oestrogen and progesterone, so some months you ovulate and some you don't. Your body tries to compensate for the lack by producing more FSH to stimulate follicle and egg production. However, this hormonal imbalance can lead to erratic and heavy periods – a build up of tissue in the endometrium (the lining of the womb) can lead to sudden flooding which is very stressful. Heavy blood loss is called perimenopausal dysfunctional uterine bleeding (DUB) and it can lead to iron deficiency, so it needs to be checked out. Your GP will also want to rule out any other possible causes such as fibroids or endometriosis.

Solutions

Make sure you carry adequate sanitary protection at all times, even if you've not had a period for a while as they can arrive unexpectedly. If you are worried about a heavy flow or have any additional symptoms, keep a note of them and speak to your GP. Maintain a balanced diet and include plenty of iron (spinach and leafy green vegetables) and try to keep up some form of exercise routine, even if it's just daily walks, as this will help relieve any pelvic cramping.

Vasomotor symptoms

Hot flushes (tropical flushes or power surges, if you prefer!)

Hot flushes are the most common symptom of perimenopause. It can be very stressful to find that your forehead is suddenly dripping and you have wet patches under your arms. According to support network Menopause Matters, they affect around 60-80% of women, with varying degrees of severity. Around 20% of women find them so disruptive that working life is affected.

When a hot flush is coming on you will typically feel a build up of heat in your face, neck and chest area which spreads out to the rest of the body. Your heart rate speeds up, you may experience dizziness and palpitations and then feel cold and shivery once it is over. You may need to change your clothes – this can be rather stressful if you are at work.

Hot flushes generally last around three to five minutes, several times a day and may continue for a couple of years during the perimenopause. They are unpredictable which can make you feel more anxious about having one and, as a consequence, they become more intense.

It isn't certain exactly why they happen but it's to do with the part of your brain that regulates temperature. Your body thinks it is hot when it isn't. In an attempt to cool you down, your blood vessels open and you sweat to release heat.

Solutions

Wear loose, natural fibres so that your skin can breathe. Layers of clothing are best because they are easy to remove. Keep your wrists and collars uncovered. Sandals and open-toed shoes enable your feet to release excess heat more quickly and a Japanese fan will help keep you cool. Carry a bottle of water with you to replenish lost fluid. It's also a good idea to look at your diet and make a few changes. Incorporate cooling foods such as salads, vegetables, fruit and smoothies, and cut back on heat-generating foods such as caffeine and spices. You could also carry a water spray containing balancing aromatherapy oils such as lavender or geranium, and regular exercise will help to reduce stress and anxiety. Practise deep breathing techniques to help you feel more in control and reduce the intensity of a flush if one does come on.

Night sweats

These typically occur around 3am-4am – you wake up with a start to find you are sweating profusely and your clothing and bedding is drenched. You get up to go to the toilet, drink some water and change your clothing. It's hard to get back to sleep because your heart is racing and you're watching the clock. Your partner is annoyed because he's now awake, shivering and the bedclothes are damp. If this scenario is happening on a regular basis, it is very stressful for you both.

Solutions

Make sure you have cotton bedding and pillowcases. Sleep naked or check out some manufacturers who sell specially designed nightwear and bedding for this purpose. The Chillow Pillow gets good reports – you slip it under your pillow at night and it reduces your body temperature, making it easier to sleep. See the help list at the back of the book for more information on getting one. You should also keep a glass of iced water by the bed.

Layer your bedding and use sheets and blankets rather than a duvet so you can toss off a layer if you get too hot. If it's putting a strain on your relationship, you could consider separate beds for part of the week. Be inventive: you could invite your partner into your boudoir on certain nights and slip off to your own bed afterwards! It's fun to do this as it takes away some of the tension that can build up when you're both struggling to get a decent night's sleep.

Breast tenderness

Fibrocystic changes (benign breast lumps) are very common during the perimenopause, affecting around 40% of women according to the charity Breakthrough Breast Cancer. Hormonal fluctuations and a drop in progesterone levels can make your breasts feel tender, sore and lumpy because the vessels and glands are swollen. This is something you've probably noticed during the menstrual cycle. Once your period arrives these symptoms tend to disappear. However, if you find a lumpy area and it doesn't disappear, then it's worth a chat with your GP to put your mind at rest. Fibrocystic changes tend to disappear after the menopause once your hormones settle down.

Solutions

Your breasts contain lymphatic tissue which is sensitive to hormonal fluctuations. The majority of breast lumps are benign and don't need to be removed as they will disappear naturally after the menopause. However, they can be uncomfortable to deal with during the perimenopause. Learning a few self-massage techniques can help. The website www.healthypages.co.uk has some excellent advice in its forums on how to do breast self massage, and therapist members suggest other useful tips, therapies and remedies that can help. Susun Weed, a leading authority on herbal medicine and women's health, has written an in-depth article called 'Breast Self Massage is Simple' for the website Suite 101 (http://www.suite101.com/article.cfm/herbalhealing/116388). It explains how to do it and which herbal oils are beneficial.

It's also important to wear a well-fitting bra, as tight bras reduce the natural lymph flow and drainage in the breast, leading to discomfort and soreness.

Insomnia

This is a common problem caused in the most part by night sweats. Being woken in the middle of the night and needing to change sheets, sanitary protection or clothing is stressful and makes it hard to get back to sleep. You don't feel rested in the morning and this can lead to exhaustion and finding it hard to cope during the day. If you are waking regularly, your body gets used to the new routine and you may find you have trouble sleeping.

Solutions

Make your bedroom as restful and inviting as possible. Avoid having any electrical equipment in the room, use a lavender silk eye mask to block out any light and try to have a bedtime routine – relax or exercise after work, read a good book, have a warm bath and go to bed at a reasonable hour. Studies have shown that the sleep gained between 11pm and 1am is deep and restful and enables our bodies to detox and regenerate fully, so try to get to bed before this time! Avoid putting the light on if you need to take a quick trip to the toilet – this stimulates the brain and tells your body it's time to get up.

If you're tossing and turning and sleep isn't happening, get up and take your mind off things. Read a good book and have some warm milk – it contains an amino acid called tryptophan which promotes relaxation and sleep. Creative thoughts usually spring to mind at odd times, so use the time to make notes on any projects you want to develop – this will help you to feel less stressed about not sleeping! For more advice on getting a good night's sleep, see Insomnia – The Essential Guide (Need2Know).

Vaginal changes

Studies have shown that although libido and orgasmic ability are maintained beyond the menopause and well into the 70s, vaginal dryness and poor lubrication is a common issue. It affects over half of postmenopausal women aged 51-60 according to a survey by Menopause Matters.

Oestrogen keeps your vagina moist, lubricated and fleshy. Small glands on the cervix and entrance to the vagina produce lubricant to enhance sex and keep the vaginal pH healthy. This also helps prevent infections from occurring.

As oestrogen levels dip, these glands don't work as efficiently and you may find it harder to lubricate, making sex feel painful and uncomfortable. The vaginal tissues become more fragile and the vagina itself shortens and narrows. In medical terms this is charmingly referred to as 'vaginal atrophy'. It sounds awful but thankfully it's not a foregone conclusion!

Solutions

You will find it takes longer to lubricate, so you will need to invest in a good quality lubricant such as Yes or Replens – this is no bad thing. Foreplay may need to take longer (sensual massage – yes, please!).

Localised oestrogen therapy in the vagina will also help. This is an alternative to taking systemic HRT which supplies the whole body with oestrogen (there's more on this in chapter 4). Speak to your GP about the options available to you.

Use it or lose it! Studies have shown that women who have regular sex have healthier vaginas and continue to lubricate. If you haven't had sex for a while, use a vibrator and lubricant regularly and it will become easier.

Vaginal and urinary infections

Another side effect of the lack of oestrogen is that the vaginal pH balance is affected. Normally oestrogen protects the urethra and vagina and keeps an acidic environment, flushing out any infections before they take hold. The most common infections to occur during perimenopause are thrush and cystitis.

Thrush

Thrush is caused by an overgrowth of yeast (Candida albicans) in the body and is quite common during your 30s and 40s. Normally yeast is carried in the body with no problems, but sometimes it can grow, giving rise to uncomfortable vaginal symptoms such as vulval inflammation, soreness and a white discharge. The vagina is usually too acidic for infections to take hold, but they are more likely to occur once oestrogen begins to decline.

Risk factors include using antibiotics, wearing tight, synthetic clothing and diabetes. Treatment options include using antifungal medication in the form of creams, tablets or pessaries.

Solutions

Try to avoid using shower gels and soaps in the area because they are perfumed and have added chemicals, causing irritation. Latex condoms and some types of lubricant can also irritate the vagina, so buy the best quality you can find. Probiotic live yoghurt is a popular remedy, as is tea tree oil bath and calendula creams. Look at your diet and cut back on any yeasty, sugary foods and alcohol.

Cystitis

Cystitis is a bladder infection that makes urinating more frequent and painful. Symptoms include painful urination, cloudy or strong-smelling urine and pain in the pelvic area. It is quite common during the menopause because low oestrogen levels make the vaginal and urinary tissues thinner and less able to withstand infection. A woman's urethra is shorter and sits close to the anal area so can easily be infected by sex or wiping from back to front when using the toilet.

Solutions

Treatment may not be necessary if it is a mild case, but if it's the first time you've had it, make sure you speak to your GP. Drink lots of water and cranberry juice to flush things through. Sit – don't squat – on the toilet so that your bladder empties properly, and always go to the toilet after having sex.

Urinary incontinence

According to the NHS, urinary incontinence affects around three million people in the UK and one in five women over 40. The two main types are stress incontinence and urge incontinence. Stress incontinence is the most common form during menopause because your muscles are weaker. You may find yourself leaking urine after coughing, laughing, sneezing or exercising. An overactive bladder causes urge incontinence – suddenly needing to go to the toilet and feeling unable to hold it back.

Solutions

There are various treatment options like regularly practising Kegel exercises to strengthen the pelvic muscles (see chapter 8). Some lifestyle changes may also be needed – being overweight and smoking puts extra strain on the bladder, and caffeine irritates the bladder and can make the problem worse.

Dr Sarah Jarvis suggests the following tips for managing stress incontinence:

- Watch your weight – being overweight increases your risk of stress incontinence.
- Veg out! Being constipated makes it worse, yet nine out of 10 women don't eat enough fibre. Increase your fruit and veg intake, as well as other sources of dietary fibre.

- Increase your water intake – you might be tempted to cut down on your fluid intake to prevent accidents. However, being dehydrated leaves you prone to bladder infections and could exacerbate the problem. Try to drink 2-21/2 litres of non-alcoholic fluid a day.
- Just a small drink for me! Alcohol acts as a diuretic which makes you pass more water, so consume it in moderation.
- Get re-acquainted with your pelvic floor – one of the most common causes of light adult incontinence is weakness of the pelvic floor, post children and when postmenopausal. Strengthening the pelvic floor can resolve this. Speak to a continence adviser via your GP or local hospital clinic for advice on the exercises.
- Be prepared – accidents will happen so use a pad such as Always Envive which has been specifically designed to provide discreet protection to keep you confident.

Aches and pains

Numbness, tingling and general aches and pains in your joints are very common during the menopause. This is caused by low levels of collagen and oestrogen, resulting in thinner, more sensitive skin. The medical term for this is paresthesia. Hot spots include the wrist, fingers, neck and shoulders.

Solutions

- Moisturise your skin well, take regular exercise and eat a diet high in essential fatty acids (fish oils, nuts and seeds) to aid blood flow.
- Avoid sitting still for too long. Self-massage and acupuncture will help relieve the symptoms.
- Eat more anti-inflammatory foods such as onions, ginger and pineapple. Herbal supplements such as black cohosh can also help – see page 52 for more information.

Other symptoms

Migraines

Studies have shown that the perimenopause can make migraines worse. Just as you may get a bad headache prior to your period starting, when hormone levels are fluctuating wildly, migraines can come on. This should settle down once you reach the menopause. In the meantime, keep a diary and monitor any foods/activities immediately before and six hours before the migraine started to see if you can pinpoint any triggers.

Weight gain

It's common to put on weight during the menopause – on average, a pound a year. This is a result of a slower metabolism and a change in hormone levels. Also, the fall in oestrogen and rise of testosterone can contribute to a change in shape – from pear to apple-shaped around the waist. You may also find that you have cravings for certain foods or just constantly feel hungry. Many women worry about HRT contributing to weight gain, but there is no evidence to back this up. You may also experience fluid retention.

Solutions include regular exercise and changes to your diet – see chapters 6 and 7 for more information.

Skin, nails and hair

A woman's skin is 10 times more sensitive than a man's, so a change in physical response and sensitivity is immediately noticeable. As we age, we lose collagen which reduces skin texture and firmness. Oestrogen makes your skin appear dewy and soft, so you may notice that your skin and hair feel dry and your nails break more easily. The best way to tackle this is to get professional advice on your hair and skincare, invest in some good quality products and include essential fatty acids in your diet.

Psychological symptoms

These are interrelated to your physical symptoms. If you aren't sleeping well due to regular night sweats, you will be feeling tired, irritable and stressed. In turn, mental stress can make physical symptoms worse.

Women going through the menopause have described the following in varying degrees of intensity:

- Mood swings.
- Sadness.
- Anxiety.
- Stress.
- Anger.
- Aggression.
- Irritability.
- Exhaustion.
- Hostility.
- Numbness.
- Unable to cope.
- Poor self image.
- Isolation.
- Panic attacks.

See chapter 7 for solutions and support.

Cognitive changes

We have oestrogen receptors all over our body including the brain, so when oestrogen levels fall, it affects our cognitive functioning. Common complaints include poor memory, lack of concentration, fogginess, panic attacks and a sense of not being on top of things intellectually.

Sexual changes

You may not feel like having sex – this is likely to be as a result of vaginal dryness and other physical changes. Low libido is often mentioned as a symptom of the menopause, but it's likely that this is connected to your thoughts and feelings about yourself, your sexual esteem and how you feel about your relationship. See chapter 8 for some solutions.

How long will these symptoms last?

Generally two to five years after they start. For some women, it may be longer or they may come and go. Even if your symptoms are mild, don't soldier on alone. It's helpful to read about other women's experiences, and talking about how you are feeling helps relieve some of the stress.

There are some excellent online support groups on forums such as Good Housekeeping, Woman and Home and Prima. Simply Hormones and The Menopause Exchange are also good places to look up information (see help list). Asking for help now will help you deal with the changes more positively and efficiently.

Checklist

- Speak to your GP or Well Woman Clinic about your symptoms.
- Keep a diary of regular occurrences and issues.
- Check out online support groups and forums.
- Keep abreast of latest research and developments.
- Deal with symptoms as they arise – don't let things drag on.

Summing Up

80% of women will experience physical, sexual and emotional symptoms during the menopause, many finding them hard to cope with. Menstrual changes, vasomotor symptoms (hot flushes, night sweats) and vaginal changes are the most common physical symptoms. These occur as a result of fluctuating hormone levels in the body and will last, on average, two to five years. You may also notice changes to your weight, skin, hair and nails which are linked to the menopause and also to ageing in general. Psychological and emotional symptoms are related to the physical and hormonal changes in your body.

It is best to deal with any symptoms as they occur rather than letting things build up. It is sensible to make some changes now to your diet, exercise routines and working life to help reduce your stress levels. Don't bottle things up. Perimenopause can be a challenging time because you may have family issues to deal with that can impact on your own health and wellbeing.

Read through online support forums such as Good Housekeeping, Prima and Woman and Home to see how other women are dealing with things. You may also find it helpful to keep a diary of your symptoms and observations to show your GP and complementary health practitioner.

Hormone Replacement Therapy (4)

What is hormone replacement therapy?

Hormone replacement therapy (HRT) is a synthetic form of your body's own natural hormones. It was developed initially to replace the loss of oestrogen and progesterone at menopause, and to relieve common symptoms such as hot flushes, night sweats and vaginal dryness. The difference between HRT and the combined contraceptive pill is that HRT is given in lower doses.

HRT has a long history and the pros and cons of use continue to be widely debated. It has been subjected to much negative press coverage since two trials were carried out in the UK and the USA which focused on its health impact.

There are over 50 types of HRT listed on the National Formulary website. The main component is synthetic oestrogen, derived from plants or equine urine (Premarin). Progestogens (synthetic progesterone) are added to the formula to induce a monthly or three-monthly bleed. This was found to be necessary after the trials showed an increase in uterine cancers among women taking the oestrogen-only formula. Understandably, since the negative reporting, HRT use has dropped significantly and women may now feel quite nervous about taking it. However, HRT has been around for 60 years or so and it's important to take a balanced view of what the research shows so far.

A brief history

The US Food and Drink Administration (FDA) approved HRT in 1941 to help relieve menopausal symptoms and to protect against long-term health issues such as osteoporosis and heart disease. The first brand was called Premarin which was developed from the urine of pregnant mares. It was thought to heal all 'women's problems' and doctors were happy to prescribe it. The first generation of HRT was quite a high dose of an oestrogen-only formula.

In the 1950s, an increase in uterine cancers was linked to the use of HRT in an oestrogen-only format. Consequently, progestogen was added to induce a bleed and protect the endometrium lining, both factors being thought to help prevent uterine cancer (Prempro being the name of one brand).

Two trials were carried out to test its safety and effectiveness:

- The Women's Heath Initiative (USA, 1993-2002)

Two trials were carried out using oestrogen-only HRT and a combined (oestrogen and progestogen) format. Results were published in 2002 and there was widespread panic after the trials were stopped due to health concerns. In the sample tested, combined HRT increased the risk of heart problems, strokes and breast cancer, but reduced the risk of fractures and colon cancer. In the oestrogen-only trial, results found no increased risk of heart attack but a higher risk of stroke and blood clots. The effect on breast cancer was inconclusive. It did not affect colorectal cancer, and it reduced the risk of fracture. (Source: The National Heart, Lung and Blood Institute, Health Information Centre.)

- The Million Women Study (UK, 1997)

This was an observational study of 1.3 million women that launched in 1997. The follow-up showed that women using HRT had a greater risk of breast cancer and a small increase in the risk of ovarian cancer. The risk of uterine cancer was linked, as with previous studies, to the use of oestrogen-only HRT in women who had not had a hysterectomy. Tibolone, a synthetic form of HRT, was also found to increase the risk of endometrial cancer.

There was panic and confusion after media reports came out stating that HRT was dangerous and that trials had been halted. Some doctors stopped prescribing HRT and many women stopped using it. However, further studies were carried out between 2004-2007 and, in retrospect, the WHI trial was found to be flawed. The subjects were much older (average age of 63 years) than the recommended age for starting HRT and some had other health issues which would have a bearing on the results. Subsequent studies on HRT use by 50-59 year old women haven't shown the same results.

Nowadays, HRT is given in the lowest possible dosage so that it is effective without risking women's health. Doctors advise that you should take it for a short period of time to relieve symptoms rather than as a long-term treatment (over 5 years). Dr Miriam Stoppard recommends trying it for three to four months initially to let the hormones get to work, then reviewing methods of delivery until you find the right one for you. This process could take up to a year until you find the right formula and dose for you, so it's not a quick fix solution. The information here is only an overview – you should talk to your GP for individual advice.

Positives of HRT

Supplementing the missing oestrogen has numerous health benefits including:

- Helping to prevent bowel cancer.
- Preventing vaginal atrophy and relieving vaginal dryness.
- Protecting and rebuilding bones.
- Protecting muscles and joints.
- Giving you more get up and go.
- Improving mood and wellbeing.

- Maintaining skin tone and moisture.
- Improving cognitive thinking and memory.
- Stopping hot flushes.

Negatives of HRT

The side effects of taking HRT are similar to those experienced in the run up to your period. In high doses, progestogen can lead to fluid retention, skin breakouts, mood swings, tender and lumpy breasts and low libido. You also have to put up with a monthly or three-monthly period which may be an inconvenience if you've been looking forward to the end of all that!

As with the contraceptive pill, some women get along with HRT and others don't. Before you dismiss it, try other types and combinations (there are lots) to find one that suits you. The most commonly reported side effects are weight gain and breast sensitivity. There is no evidence to show that it causes weight gain and, as Norma Goldman of The Menopause Exchange points out, any weight gain is most likely to be age-related. The best way to avoid this is to increase exercise and keep an eye on your diet.

Different types of HRT

There are three main types:

- Oestrogen-only – this is for women who have had a hysterectomy and don't need progestogen to protect the lining of the womb from over-stimulation.
- Cyclical/sequential – suitable for women who are still menstruating. You can opt for a monthly bleed or a three-monthly bleed pattern. It is a combination of oestrogen and progestogen.
- Continuous (period-free) – a continuous combination of oestrogen and progestogen for postmenopausal women. You won't have a period with this type of HRT.

How to take it

Following is a list of ways HRT can be administered.

- Tablets (oral or vaginal).
- Skin patches, creams, gels or nasal spray.
- An implant – small pellets beneath the skin.
- Vaginal ring.

It's helpful to read up on the different delivery methods and explore the pros and cons of each to help you make the right choice. Tablets are most commonly prescribed, however they tend to be a slightly stronger dose because they have to go through the liver which, unfortunately, raises the risk of gallstones and liver damage.

Patches, creams and gels are a newer form of delivery and are considered to be superior because they go directly into the bloodstream. They may produce fewer side effects as the dose is slightly lower. However, they can be more expensive.

Implants can be left in place for up to six months and once they are in you can forget about them. Vaginal creams, tablets and rings work locally, increasing oestrogen levels in the vagina only. This is beneficial if you are experiencing painful sex due to dry vaginal tissues but aren't having severe hot flushes.

SERMS (selective estrogen receptor modulators)

This is a new form of HRT which is a little bit more sophisticated. Instead of supplying the whole body with oestrogen, it targets receptors in the brain and body, supplying you with oestrogen where you need it most. Trials to date have been encouraging, showing it has protective effects against osteoporosis and heart disease. Tamoxifen and Raloxifene are two main types.

Alternatives to HRT (on prescription)

- The combined contraceptive pill may be offered as an alternative to HRT, but it contains higher doses of oestrogen and progestogen. It's not suitable for all women.
- Tibolone is a synthetic steroid that contains oestrogen and progestogen in one formula.
- Clonidine/Dixarit – a prescription drug for migraines and high blood pressure. It can help reduce hot flushes and night sweats.

Bio-identical hormones – the future of HRT

If you're not happy with the 'one-size-fits-all' approach of conventional HRT, you may want to consider trying bio-identical hormones. These are considered by many to be the future of HRT. They contain the same chemical structure as our body's own hormones so are thought to be safer, easier to metabolise and less likely to cause side effects. They are made from plant sources – a substance called diosgenin found in wild yams. They work by combining bio-identical oestrogen with natural progesterone and, if required, testosterone supplements. Dr John Moran and Dr Marion Gluck both work extensively in this field providing bespoke HRT treatments for women.

US Author Suzanne Somers has written extensively about the positive effects of bio-identical hormones on her menopause in her book The Sexy Years. Dr Shirley Bond and Anna Rushton also discuss it in their book Natural Progesterone.

Checklist

- Do you know about the different types of HRT and delivery methods?
- Make an appointment to speak to your GP/gynaecologist about your options for HRT.
- Talk to your GP for further information and advice. The information contained here is only an overview – your GP will be able to give you professional medical advice.

Summing Up

There are over 50 types of HRT and it's not a case of one-size-fits-all. If you don't get along with the first formula you try, ask your GP for another type.

The initial trials for HRT which linked it to breast cancer and other health issues were found to be flawed and would not be permitted now under the same conditions.

HRT is an effective treatment for most menopausal symptoms. The national guidelines now state it should be delivered in a low dose for short-term use.

Bio-identical hormones are a very popular option. They contain the same chemical structure as your body's own so are safer, easier to metabolise and have fewer side effects. In a debate at this year's European Menopause Conference, the general feeling was that they are a very positive step.

Complementary and Alternative Medicine (CAM) (5)

What is CAM?

Complementary and Alternative Medicine (CAM) works alongside conventional medicine to help heal the body. The NHS Directory of Complementary and Alternative Practitioners has further information on the different types of therapy available and how they work. The House of Lords Science and Technical Committee's report on complementary therapies divides them into three distinct groups:

- Group 1 – includes those therapies that have a diagnostic approach such as osteopathy and chiropractic. These have been regulated by Acts of Parliament. It also includes acupuncture, herbal medicine and homeopathy.
- Group 2 – includes complementary therapies which aren't diagnostic in approach: bodywork, aromatherapy, Alexander technique, counselling, hypnotherapy, healing, reflexology and shiatsu.
- Group 3 – includes therapies that have their own philosophies and don't follow the approach of conventional medicine. This includes Ayurveda and traditional Chinese medicine.

This chapter gives an overview of therapies that have been found useful for treating menopausal symptoms, either anecdotally or via scientific studies where possible. If you are considering using CAM, find a practitioner via a regulatory body for that particular therapy.

Get advice from your GP and speak to them about different approaches as some, such as homeopathy and acupuncture, may be available in certain cases on the NHS.

Using CAM is a positive step in helping your body to correct its own hormonal balance. It will also help you de-stress and find some valuable 'me time' which is healing in itself!

Acupuncture

Acupuncture is divided into two types: traditional Chinese which dates back 2,000 years, and Western acupuncture which was recently developed and is based on conventional medicine. Fine needles are inserted into the skin to stimulate our meridians (energy centres) to aid blood circulation and release muscular tensions. It acts as a release and is surprisingly gentle and relaxing to receive. It can also help to regulate changes in the hormonal system throughout the menopause. A therapist will take a detailed medical history, note any symptoms and use the needles accordingly to relieve pain and release areas of tension.

Low levels of oestrogen during the menopause are linked to poor functioning of the parts of the brain that govern our hormones and changes in the central nervous system (the brain and spinal cord). Acupuncture corrects this poor functioning (imbalance) and increases endorphins via the peripheral nervous system. A 2004 Swedish study found that it decreased hot flushes by 83% in those tested. Contact the British Society of Acupuncture for further details (see help list).

Alexander technique

Australian Frederick Matthias Alexander developed the Alexander technique in the 1890s. It teaches you the principles of good posture (head, neck and back alignment) and breathing techniques to put less stress on the body and improve physical and mental performance. Studies have found that it can improve balance and reduce the risk of falls in later life. It can also help reduce high blood pressure and cardiovascular problems, tension-related sexual disorders and migraines. Studies in 1985 and 1992 showed improvement in lung capacity and deeper, slower breathing which can help reduce the impact of hot flushes. Contact the Society of Alexander Technique for further details (see help list).

Aromatherapy

Aromatherapy uses plant oils to prevent and treat different symptoms. It has a long history of use, dating back thousands of years. There are various ways you can use it: via inhalation, in the bath, during massage or by making your own body creams. The plant oils have an immediate and powerful effect on the senses, sending messages to the limbic system, the part of the brain that controls our emotions. This system helps to regulate our hormonal system, so, in effect, oils can help rebalance your hormones during the perimenopause. Aromatherapy can help relieve stress, tension, allow an emotional release and relieve insomnia, headaches and PMT.

Aromatherapy oils for the menopause

'Florals are great for dealing with the emotions,' says Carol Preen, Vice Chair of the Allied Aromatherapy Practitioners' Association (AAPA) and senior lecturer in aromatherapy at Morley College, London. 'Rose is the queen of oils and good for treating female problems. It is very concentrated, so you only need one drop at a time (it takes 30 roses to make one drop of oil!). Rose is a purifier and regulator, so it helps to regulate the menstrual cycle and reduce heavy periods. It is also good for the nerves if you are feeling uptight and anxious. It works as an antidepressant, creating a positive feeling and lightness of heart. It helps to release the hormone dopamine which puts us in a good mood.'

- Geranium helps to balance the adrenal cortex which produces androgens (male sex hormones). It is also good for inflammation and can help reduce fluid retention. It is an all over tonic – it acts as an antidepressant and stress reducer.

- Frankincense is good for dealing with emotions. It is a uterine tonic so can help ease heavy periods and rebalance the reproductive system. It is calming and good for anxiety and dark moods.

For a little extra help getting through the day, add a few drops of your chosen oil to a small carrier bottle and sniff throughout the day (combine with a base oil such as sweet almond).

Ayurveda

Ayurveda is the Sanskrit word for 'life knowledge'. It is often referred to as the 'science of life' and is an ancient Indian system of healthcare dating back around 3500 years. Practitioners work alongside conventional doctors to help treat patients holistically and will draw up a treatment plan based on dietary advice, exercise and herbal medicines. It works on the principle that we have a mixture of energies in the body, Vata, Pitta and Kapha, which need to be rebalanced for optimum health. It can help treat insomnia, headaches, tension and anxiety, high blood pressure and blood sugar imbalance. Contact the Ayurveda Association for further details (see help list).

Bach Flower Remedies

These are based on the pioneering work of Harley Street doctor Edward Bach in the 1930s. He formulated 38 flower remedies to treat specific emotions, promoting the idea that physical health was related to mental health. The seven emotional groups which form the basis for the remedies are as follows:

- Fear.
- Loneliness.
- Not being in the present moment.
- Despair.
- Uncertainty.

- Over-sensitivity.
- Over-caring for others.

Bach Rescue Remedy is a combination of five original flower essences: Rock Rose, Impatiens, Clematis, Star of Bethlehem and Cherry Plum to help relieve stress and tension so that you can get through the day. The Bach Centre has further advice and links to practitioners (see help list).

Bowen technique

Australian Tom Bowen developed the Bowen technique in the 1950s. 'Simply stated, the Bowen technique resets the body to heal itself. It creates a deep sense of relaxation, and healing seems to occur by affecting the body's autonomic nervous system, which creates homeostasis at the cellular level', says European College of Bowen Studies teacher and practitioner Jo Lunn. 'It is a very gentle technique and rolling type moves are performed on the skin over the connective tissue. It may be done through light clothing and no oil or lotion is used. There are frequent, important pauses between these moves, which give the body time to benefit from each set. By combining moves, both in placement and in combination, the practitioner is able to address the body as a whole or target a specific problem. A unique tool of the Bowen practitioner is "tissue tension sense", meaning that a practitioner is able to discern stress build-up in muscle groups and then utilise Bowen moves to release tension.'

Counselling

WPF Therapy (formerly Westminster Pastoral Foundation), a London-based charity, runs a project to help you manage the life changes that occur when you reach 50. They point out that midlife can be tough and counselling in this form can help you to deal with the emotional aspects of reaching the menopause. This is just as important as dealing with the physical changes. Contact the charity for further details (see help list).

Herbal medicine

Western herbal medicine uses plant remedies as a form of healing. It takes a holistic approach, looking at an individual's symptoms to determine the appropriate treatment. Contact a qualified herbalist for individual assessment and treatment for your particular symptoms. This will generally be stronger and more effective than any over-the-counter remedies you can buy. Popular hormonal regulating herbs for menopause include the following:

- Black cohosh – used by native Americans for years, this is said to help relieve hot flushes, sweats and vaginal dryness. There is a suggested link to liver damage but the evidence is inconclusive; talk to your GP before taking it or if you have any concerns. It should not be used if you have any existing health issues such as stroke, high blood pressure, cancer or certain allergies. If you decide to try it, buy a reputable, quality brand to ensure purity, as this can be an issue. Better still, consult a qualified medical herbalist who can tailor it to your specific symptoms.
- Agnus castus – works on the pituitary gland to balance hormones, relieve hot flushes and improve libido.
- Dong quai – an all-over female tonic. It balances the reproductive system, boosts energy levels, increases circulation and protects muscles, bones and joints.
- Ginkgo biloba – improves memory and concentration by stimulating blood circulation.

Contact the National Institute of Medical Herbalists for further details (see help list).

Homeopathy

Homeopathy involves using minute doses of plant, animal and mineral remedies to treat symptoms and stimulate recovery. Samuel Hahnemann, a German pharmacist, founded it in the 19th century. There are five homeopathic hospitals on the NHS, so it's worth speaking to your GP about homeopathy. It can help with hot flushes, night sweats, tiredness, anxiety, insomnia and headaches. One study at the NHS Well Woman Clinic in Sheffield reported that 81% of 102 patients assessed reported an improvement in menopausal symptoms after using homeopathy. Contact the Society of Homeopaths for further details (see help list).

Hypnotherapy

Hypnotherapy is a powerful relaxation technique that works on the subconscious mind to release negative thought patterns. It can help with low self-esteem, sexual issues, addictions, panic attacks, depression and stress. Different methods are used to achieve this including voice, music and imagery. Hypnotherapist Georgia Foster has written several books on the subject and has developed CDs to use at home for self-hypnosis and relaxation. See her website www.georgiafoster.com for more information.

Reflexology

Reflexology works on trigger points in the feet and hands to stimulate release and healing in corresponding organs in the body. 'It works on the parasympathetic nervous system to calm us down', says Glenys Underwood, a Fellow of the Association of Reflexologists and founder of the Caritas School of Reflexology in Lincolnshire. 'It goes hand in hand with women's problems and is invaluable during the menopause.' The big toe and ankle area are related to the reproductive and endocrine systems. If an organ is under pressure, you will feel tenderness in the related area on your foot. The heel of the foot is linked to the pelvic area, so work here can help with other symptoms of menopause such as painful sex.

The British Menopause Society Consensus

In response to the increased interest and awareness of CAM to aid menopausal symptoms, the British Menopause Society issued a consensus statement in 2007 which is outlined below.

'The British Menopause Society Council aims to aid health professionals to inform and advise women about the menopause. This guidance regarding alternative and complementary therapies is in response to the increased use of these strategies by women who believe them to be safer and more "natural". The choice is confusing. Evidence from randomised trials that alternative and complementary therapies improve menopausal symptoms or have the same benefits as HRT is poor.

A major concern is interaction with other treatments, with potentially fatal consequences. Some preparations may contain estrogenic compounds, and this is a concern for women with hormone-dependent diseases such as breast cancer. Concern also exists about the quality control of production. While a European Union Directive on traditional herbal medicinal products was implemented in October 2005 in the UK, this will not cover products bought by women outside Europe.'

So do your research. Speak to friends and family and ask for recommendations. Check a therapist's credentials and if you do go ahead with treatments, take them slowly and one at a time. That way you can monitor how effective they are.

Checklist

- What type of complementary therapies would you like to try?
- What is best suited to your particular symptoms?
- Are you taking any other medication that could impact on the effectiveness of a therapy?
- Does your GP have any recommendations?
- Start keeping a diary of any treatments you've tried to monitor effectiveness.

Summing Up

CAM works alongside conventional medicine to help heal the body. It is divided into three distinct groups: therapies such as osteopathy which have a diagnostic approach, complementary therapies such as bodywork which aren't diagnostic and therapies such as Ayurveda which have their own history and philosophy.

Certain therapies may be available on the NHS so it's worth speaking to your GP if there is something specific you would like to try. By asking your GP, you can make sure that it doesn't interfere with current medication.

The BMS issued a consensus statement in 2007, with the aim of informing and advising women about the menopause. This is shown on their website (www.thebms.org.uk) and states that a major concern with using CAM is interaction with other treatments and the quality control of production. Exercise caution and do your research about different therapies and treatments. Always consult a qualified practitioner and get advice from your GP. Complementary therapists are regulated by a founding body which should be your first port of call for advice and recommendation.

Nutrition and the Menopause (6)

There are two camps when it comes to treating the menopause: those who think it is a hormonal deficiency that needs to be treated with drugs (HRT) and those, such as nutritionist and author Marilyn Glenville, who advocate the natural approach: using diet to ease your way through the menopause. Her book New, Natural Alternatives to HRT explores this in detail.

This chapter looks at ways to alter your diet and detox your body to improve menopausal symptoms. As nutritional therapist Julie G Silver suggests, regular menstruation is your body's natural way of detoxing, so when this stops we need to find other ways to detox to maintain our health.

What is a balanced diet?

A balanced diet incorporates foods from the five major food groups.

Carbohydrates

These should form a third of your diet. They can be found in bread, pasta, potatoes, cereals and rice. Opt for complex carbs (eg, brown bread and pasta) for a higher fibre count. Simple carbs (eg, white bread and sugar) can make hot flushes worse. Foods high in fibre help the body to expel toxins.

Protein

Protein should amount to a fifth of your diet. It protects and repairs your body, and protein-rich foods also contain other essential vitamins and minerals. Eggs, meat, fish, beans, tofu, soya and nuts are all good sources of protein. Tryptophan is an amino acid found in proteins such as milk, cheese and eggs and has been found to raise serotonin levels, boosting mood and promoting sleep.

Fruit and vegetables

High in vitamins and minerals, fruit and vegetables keep your hair, skin and nails healthy and can help prevent disease. The government guidelines recommend five portions of fruit and vegetables a day. Try to buy organic varieties whenever possible.

Dairy

Dairy foods are rich in calcium and help to protect your bones and teeth. Aim for 1000mg a day (see opposite for examples). Cheese, yoghurts, milk (dairy and soya), spinach, tinned fish and sesame seeds are good sources.

Good fats

Fats are divided into various groups (see the two 'good fats' below). You need to watch your intake of saturated fats (fats that solidify at room temperature and are from animal sources) including butter, cream, pastries, cakes and fried foods. Limit these to 20g a day. This is the equivalent of a cheese sandwich and two slices of toast with butter, both of which contain around 10g of saturated fat each. Foods that are high in saturated fat contain more than 5g of saturated fat per 100g.

- Unsaturated fats – found in vegetable oil, avocados, nuts, seeds and oily fish. They can help to reduce cholesterol and are far better for you than saturated fats.

- Monounsaturated fats – these are found in olive oil, hummous and nuts containing omegas 3 and 6. This fat type helps to keep your joints healthy, so try to make these the dominant part of your fat intake.

Source: NHS Choices.

Tips for a healthy diet during the menopause

- Drink more water – aim for one to two litres a day. If you're suffering from hot flushes and night sweats, it's important to replenish missing fluid.
- Cut down on caffeine – coffee, tea and chocolate all stimulate the central nervous system. Caffeine dehydrates the body and more than two or three cups of coffee a day increases anxiety levels and affects sleeping habits. A high intake has been linked to hot flushes, fibrocystic changes to the breast and menstrual cramping.
- Cut down on any alcohol you drink – alcohol can trigger hot flushes and stops your body from absorbing nutrients properly. It also contributes to weight gain.
- Increase your calcium intake – you will need to counteract bone loss after the menopause. The National Osteoporosis Society recommends a daily intake of around 1000mg a day. This is equivalent to half a pint of semi-skimmed or soya milk, a dairy rich meal (cheesy pasta or sandwich), breakfast cereal and a low fat yoghurt. Leafy green vegetables, tinned fish such as sardines and sesame seeds are also rich in calcium. Opt for reduced fat dairy products if you want to keep an eye on your saturated fat intake.
- Quit smoking – studies have shown that smokers reach the menopause two years earlier. It's thought that nicotine lowers oestrogen levels and prevents the stimulation of follicles and in turn, ovulation. Smoking is ageing, dulls the skin, makes hot flushes worse and makes exercise and breathing hard work – what more incentive do you need to quit?

Harley Street dietician, author and broadcaster Nigel Denby points out that it's not necessary to radically overhaul your diet during menopause. This is daunting and difficult to maintain. He recommends making two or three small changes gradually and seeing them through.

Weight gain at menopause

Dr Jane Johnston points out that every year over the age of 40 our basal metabolic rate (the rate at which we burn off calories) slows down. So, if you continue to follow your usual eating and exercise habits, you will put on a pound a year. We also lose muscle mass and begin to store fat for later (our bodies want to preserve our oestrogen stores for as long as possible!). Your shape may also change from pear-like curves to an apple-shaped midriff. This is connected to testosterone production which can rise during the perimenopause.

However, it's not all bad news. As broadcaster and Woman's Hour presenter Jenni Murray points out in her book Is it Me, or is it Hot in Here?, excessive dieting isn't a good idea. It deprives the body of essential nutrients. Carrying a little extra weight prolongs our body's production of oestrogen, keeping us healthy and younger-looking for longer, as well as maintaining its other protective effects. To maintain a healthy weight and muscle mass eat small, healthy meals regularly to maintain blood sugar levels and exercise for at least 20 minutes a day, including some weight-bearing and resistance training. There are more exercise tips in the next chapter.

Your weekly diet for menopause

Nutritionist and natural health and stress management consultant Julie G Silver recommends the following weekly diet plan:

‘Go for a diet rich in wholegrains such as quinoa, millet, brown rice or wheat free pasta or noodles if you haven’t got the time to make a grain. Serve with fresh or tinned salmon, mackerel, organic chicken or organic free-range eggs. If you are vegetarian use beans, lentils, tofu or tempeh. Tofu and tempeh contain phytoestrogens (naturally ocurring plant compounds that mimic the role of oestrogen in the body) which are ideal for menopausal symptoms and can help reduce the risk of breast cancer. Serve with lots of fresh vegetables and salad. Cabbage, kale, broccoli, sprouts and cauliflower are all rich in phytonutrients (nutrients obtained from plants which help the body to function well).

‘Sea vegetables such as arame, nori and kombu can be used in cooking to enhance minerals and help balance hormones but need to be introduced slowly. Kelp can be taken as a supplement – you’ll find it in Total Nutrition Superfood, available from Better You.

‘Pumpkin, sunflower seeds, hemp seeds and nuts such as almonds, hazelnuts and walnuts are a good source of protein and contain magnesium, iron, zinc, vitamin E and essential fatty acids. A small handful of seeds and nuts a day is a good way to get your quota of essential fats and minerals.

‘Linseeds (flaxseeds) help to alleviate menopausal symptoms as they help rebalance prostaglandins. They have many qualities including alleviating adverse symptoms of menopause. I would recommend milled flaxseeds which you can find in a health shop or supermarket. Sprinkle a dessertspoon on your breakfast cereal or add to water.

‘Aim for one to two portions of oily fish per week to increase your levels of essential fatty acids.

‘Avoid caffeine, which affects the adrenal glands in a negative way. Eat regularly to keep your blood sugar levels balanced and try to avoid sugary foods. Too much fruit can elevate your blood sugar levels. Foods that contain hydrogenated fats, artificial colours and preservatives and sweeteners are also detrimental to your health.’

Beneficial nutrients include Maca which can be used as an alternative to HRT. It stimulates and regulates the endocrine system, supports the immune system, increases energy and libido and is rich in calcium, magnesium, phosphorus and iron as well as other trace minerals and B vitamins. The calcium and magnesium are absorbable and have been used successfully to prevent and reverse osteoporosis.

Brazilian Ginseng contains a complete spectrum of vitamins, trace minerals and amino acids. It also contains a plant sterol called stigmasterol which is a good alternative to HRT as it is a precursor to oestrogen, helping the body to maintain its own levels naturally.

Linda Kearns' menopause cake

Linda Kearns came up with the idea of a HRT-alternative cake during her menopause after being prescribed HRT and wanting to find a more natural way of treating her symptoms. She developed a cake that is high in phytoestrogens that have been found to be beneficial in treating menopausal symptoms. The recipe for the cake has been published so you can bake your own version or buy it online from www.bake-it.com.

The cake contains soya flour, soya milk, pumpkin seeds, raisins, linseeds, sesame seeds, nuts, dried fruit and spices to taste. Nutritionist Marilyn Glenville believes it could be effective and points to studies that show that eating soya over a two-week period helped to get rid of hot flushes.

Linda has published a book Eat To Beat Menopause: Over 100 Recipes to Help You Overcome the Symptoms of Menopause. The recipes included contain phystoestrogens and calcium. Some women say it can be beneficial to switch to a diet low in dairy and high in phytoestrogens during the perimenopause.

Dietary supplements

There are hundreds of dietary supplements for the menopause and it can be quite daunting deciding what to take, not to mention expensive. If you have read press reports about a particular product being useful and want to get a second opinion, it's worth speaking to your GP, pharmacist or contacting The Menopause Exchange for advice. The founder of The Menopause Exchange, Norma Goldman, suggests that natural supplements are useful for women who don't want to/can't take HRT. Typical ingredients include hops which are a sedative and isoflavones which can help reduce symptoms. You can buy online from reputable suppliers such as the Organic Pharmacy or Victoria Health who advise on the products they sell. Popular supplements for menopause include VitalWOMAN, Estroven, Red Clover, Femergy and Menopace.

Superfood: phytoestrogens

Phytoestrogens have been widely studied and can help relieve certain symptoms as well as rebalance your hormones.

Much has been made of the fact that the Japanese don't have a word for 'hot flushes', let alone experience them – well, if they do, they keep it quiet! They also have very low rates of breast cancer, and both of these facts have been attributed to their diet which is naturally high in phytoestrogens and low in animal fats. Studies have shown that Japanese women who moved to the west and adopted a normal Western diet suffered typical menopausal symptoms. Further research into the effects of phytoestrogens on the menopause is ongoing.

There are two types of phytoestrogens:

- Lignans – found in high fibre foods, wheat bran, rye, fruit and vegetables, flaxseed and sunflower.
- Isoflavones – genistein and daidsein have been studied and found to help reduce hot flushes. Good food sources include soya products, tofu, beans, pulses and chickpeas (hummous).

Checklist

- Keep a food and drink diary for a week to see if you can identify anything that is aggravating hot flushes. Common culprits include spicy foods, caffeine and alcohol.
- Shop ahead and stock up on recommended foods. Have a go at baking your own menopause cake.
- Buy a menopausal recipe book for inspiration and new ideas such as Eat To Beat Menopause: Over 100 Recipes to Help You Overcome the Symptoms of Menopause by Linda Kearns.

Summing Up

Good nutrition can have a huge impact on your wellbeing and can improve certain menopausal symptoms such as hot flushes and night sweats, as well as protecting your health in the long term. Regular menstruation is your body's way of detoxing naturally, so when this slows down and stops, we need to find other ways to detox to maintain our health.

A balanced diet incorporates foods from the major five groups: carbohydrates, protein, dairy, fruit and veg, and good fats. Try and include five portions of fruit and veg a day and go for complex carbs (brown bread, rice and pasta) over white flour to help you feel energised and full for longer. It's important to maintain a healthy body mass index (BMI) as this will help your body to cope with physical changes more efficiently, as well as protecting your health in the long-term. To work this out you need to know your height and weight. Visit www.bbc.co.uk/healthy/healthy_living/your_weight/bmiimperial_index.shtml for an online BMI calculator. BMI measurements are classified into four groups: underweight (below 18.5), ideal weight (18.5-25), overweight (25-30) and obese (30-40).

Being a healthy weight for your height lowers your risk of developing diabetes, reduces blood pressure and promotes high energy levels.

Phytoestrogens, substances found in plants (soya, linseed), have been widely studied for their beneficial effects on menopausal symptoms and can help reduce hot flushes. Soya is a good substitute for everyday dairy products.

There are various menopausal supplements and some are more effective than others. If you are considering taking a nutritional supplement, it may be worth speaking to a qualified herbalist for an individual prescription that targets your specific symptoms.

Exercise and Lifestyle Changes (7)

It is important to keep up a regular exercise routine throughout life for brain and body function. During the menopause various physical changes are occurring and you may need to adapt your current exercise routine to account for this. Exercise during the menopause and beyond needs to incorporate aerobic exercise, flexibility and strength/resistance training. Experts recommend aiming for up to an hour a day, three to five times a week, for optimum health.

This isn't as time consuming as it sounds. It doesn't have to be all at once – several, shorter bursts of exercise (brisk walking, housework, walking up the stairs, shopping!) all count towards it. Try to increase your physical activity during a normal day: take the stairs instead of the lift, walk or cycle to work or go for a brisk walk at lunchtime. You could even invest in a pedometer to track your steps throughout the day. A gradual accumulation of exercise will have a big impact on your fitness levels and how alert you feel.

Health benefits of regular exercise

- Improves your memory and cognitive thinking.
- Reduces the frequency and severity of hot flushes.
- Produces endorphins which put you in a positive frame of mind.
- Aids detox and enables your body to get rid of waste more quickly.
- Improves skin tone and appearance.
- Reduces stress levels.
- Increases bone density to protect against osteoporosis.
- Helps you to sleep better.
- Improves self-esteem and body image.

Why we put on weight during the menopause

There are various reasons for this. As we get older, our metabolism slows down and we lose muscle tone which means the rate at which we burn fat is slower. Sweet food cravings and an increase in appetite are also common during perimenopause due to fluctuating hormones – this can contribute to weight gain over time.

Researchers at Oregon Health and Science University, USA, have established a link between the menopause and weight gain. They studied 47 monkeys, 19 of which had their ovaries removed (the other 28 were observed as a placebo group). They found that the drop in hormones in the monkeys without ovaries led to a 67% increase in food intake and 5% increase in weight gain.

A study published in the Journal of the North American Menopause Society, 1995 (Vol 2, No 4, pp 201-9), found that lower ovarian hormonal production has an impact on how quickly we metabolise food. The researchers concluded that regular exercise has as big an impact on health and wellbeing as HRT. It is good for our mental health and protects against osteoporosis and heart disease.

Weight gain around this time isn't inevitable. You simply need to make a few minor changes to your diet and exercise routine and you will be in better shape than ever. Regular exercise and a good diet will help reduce the severity of menopausal symptoms.

Exercise through your menopause

Opposite, Lucy Wyndham-Read, an online fitness coach, suggests a couple of exercise routines that you can do at home and outdoors to maximise bone strength, flexibility and muscle tone.

'The important thing with exercise is that it has to be consistent and should really be done at least three times a week,' Lucy advises. 'With busy lifestyles it can be a challenge to find time to schedule in a gym visit. A great alternative is to bring the gym to your front room. Your exercise routine should consist of some form of aerobic activity such as walking, jogging, swimming, cycling or dancing. The other important form of exercise is strength training as this keeps your bones strong so can help prevent osteoporosis. This naturally increases your metabolic rate so you burn more calories on a daily basis. The key thing is finding an activity you love so you are more likely to stick with it.'

Your home circuit

You will need a mat or towel, a clock with a second hand and two bottles of water or dumbbells.

Write the name of each of the exercises below on a piece of paper and set up the five stations in a circle.

Start with a two minute warm up by marching on the spot then move to station number one. Do the exercise for one minute then jog or march for one minute before moving straight on to the next station. After you reach your last station, march on the spot for two minutes as you cool down. You can repeat the circuit again if you want to.

Station 1: The squat

Stand with your feet hip width distance apart, arms bent at sides and tummy pulled in tight. Bend your knees and push your buttocks back as if you were going to sit in a chair, lowering until thighs are parallel to the ground. Repeat this move for one minute.

Station 2: The chest toner

Stand with good posture, feet hip width distance apart and knees slightly bent. Lift your arms so your elbows are bent at a 90-degree angle to the shoulder. Press your elbows, forearms and hands together. Keeping your elbows high, lift your hands up towards the ceiling. Keep your forearms pressed together. Slowly lower your elbows back to the start position (if you allow them to drop too low it will reduce the effectiveness of the exercise). Repeat this move for one minute.

Station 3: The lunge

Stand with your feet hip width apart and arms at your side with palms facing inwards. Take one long step forward and bend both knees so the front knee is aligned with the ankle and the back heel is slightly lifted. Don't allow your back knee to touch the floor as you push yourself back up. Repeat on the other leg. Do this for one minute.

Station 4: The back and shoulder toner

Stand with good posture, holding water bottles or dumbbells in both hands. Keep your elbows tucked into your sides, your forearms at a 90-degree angle and your hands shoulder width distance apart. Keeping your elbows close to your sides, move your hands out to the side while keeping your elbows tucked in. This is a small movement but you will feel it working your upper back. Keep your tummy muscles pulled in and your abdominals tight. Do this for one minute.

Station 5: The abdominal toner

Lie face up with your feet flat and arms out by your side on either your mat or towel. Slowly lift your head and shoulders off the ground and keep your tummy muscles pulled in tight. Your elbows and chin should be level. Lower and repeat. Repeat this move for one minute.

Aim to do this indoor circuit three times a week and always remember to stretch after each workout.

Get toned in the great outdoors

Exercising outdoors is a great way of reducing stress and depression and the fresh air can really increase your energy levels. If you are exercising between 11am-3pm, avoid being in direct sunlight, make sure you drink plenty of water and top up the sunscreen. In the winter, always wear plenty of layers and bright, reflective clothing.

This circuit will improve your fitness, increase bone density, raise your ability to burn calories, reduce depression and help to reduce hot flushes. It will also tone and sculpt your body.

Outdoor circuit

Start off with a 10 minute brisk walk, add the three exercises below and finish off with another 10 minute brisk walk.

Upper arm toner

Sit on a bench and have your hands by your bottom with your fingers facing you. Keep your knees bent and both feet flat on the floor. Slowly lower your body off the bench, keeping your back straight and bending through the elbows. Lower several inches then push back up. Aim to do this 10-20 times.

Chest toner

Stand six inches away from a wide tree. Place your hands shoulder width distance apart and at chest height, with your arms fully straightened. Slowly lower your upper body towards the tree, hold and then push back up. Aim to do this 10-20 times.

Lower body toner

Use a low bench or a step. Simply step up and down, keeping your back straight and your abdominals pulled in tight. Do 20 steps leading with one leg and then switch to the other leg.

Aim to do this circuit three times a week. Always remember to stretch after your workout.

Self-esteem and time for you

The menopause is a transition to the next stage of your life. If you've been busy raising children, developing a relationship and working full time, you may feel it's time to make some changes. It's important to look after your health and wellbeing and to give yourself some valuable 'red tent' time, as psychotherapist and life coach Dr Daphne Stevens describes it. By this she means taking stock of your life, creating space to meditate and relax, developing your own interests and relationships, setting new goals and becoming part of your community.

Dr Stevens conducts retreats for women going through the menopause based on the ideas behind Anita Diamant's best-selling book The Red Tent which is a celebration of womanhood. Finding retreats and workshops will increase your social networks and help you to focus on your spiritual needs. Think about what experiences you've had, what you have to offer younger women and how you can be a role model and mentor to those who need some guidance and direction.

If you are struggling with a sense of identity and wondering what to focus on next, it can be helpful to talk to a counsellor about your feelings. WPF is a charity based in London that runs courses for women over 50 to help them address life issues. For their contact details see the help list.

Life coaching

Life coaching can help you work out what you want to do next and how you are going to get there. You may be mulling over a new business idea and feel unsure about how to get started. Look for a coach who has an interest in your field. They will have useful information and contacts to help you get started. Talking regularly and setting goals with someone who is open and motivated will help you move forward quickly. It's surprising how we can talk ourselves down or think up reasons why we shouldn't do something. A life coach can help you to keep things in perspective.

‘There may appear to be few positives about reaching the menopause at first,’ says life coach Carol Ann Rice (The Real Coaching Co), ‘however, it is a time of change. Perhaps you’re becoming more independent again after having children. You could be building a new career or taking up new interests. Hopefully you will have more financial support and can invest in the things you’ve always wanted to do. You can start to think about being more responsibly selfish. You may be grieving about losing your youth, but you may find it is a relief not to be objectified by men anymore. You may find that your relationships with men improve. Maintaining a sexual image is a burden and can be quite exhausting! You may feel more relaxed about walking down the street anonymously and enjoy the freedom that comes with that. I saw a girl the other day tottering down the street in six-inch heels. She could barely walk and looked most uncomfortable. I thought to myself, thank goodness I don’t have to put myself through that anymore!’

Carol suggests the following tips for building self-esteem and making the best of yourself:

- Invest in a few classic outfits and accessorise with big, chunky jewellery to keep your style fresh.
- Start clubs in your local area or get communities together via the Internet. Have a great time forming alliances. Women in Business is one such organisation that is worth belonging to.
- Think about how you can be a role model for younger women. It will give you a great deal of satisfaction to share your knowledge and skills with women in their 20s which will help them move forward.
- Try to be open minded about new music charts and the latest films – you may be pleasantly surprised!

- Look around you. There are many amazing women out there: Jo Wood, Oprah Winfrey, Joanna Lumley, Vivienne Westwood, Maya Angelou – you have more power than ever. You are less self-conscious and less concerned with seeking the perfect body. There is a wonderful freedom in that. Self-acceptance is a very peaceful state to be in. This is your time now so make the most of it.

Checklist

- Find out about support networks in your local area – or consider starting your own group.
- Check out charities that offer counselling and courses.
- Keep the levels of communication wide – speak to your GP and family about how you are feeling.
- Cut out roles and responsibilities that drain your energy. Spend time around people and things that lift your spirits.
- Put some exercise time in the diary for the next few weeks and follow it through. Is there someone who could 'buddy' you so you can motivate each other?
- Make a list of the things you'd like to change about yourself – a new haircut, wardrobe and also ways of developing your spiritual interests.

Summing Up

It is important to keep up a regular exercise routine throughout life for optimum brain and body function. Exercise during the menopause and beyond needs to incorporate aerobic exercise, flexibility and strength and resistance training. Experts recommend aiming for up to an hour a day, three to five times a week for optimum health. The best way to achieve this is to increase your physical activity throughout the day and make small changes to your routine. This will have a big impact on your fitness levels and how alert you feel.

As we age, we tend to gain weight due to a slow down in our metabolism and the rate at which we burn fat. Fluctuating hormone levels can also trigger sweet cravings and can impact how quickly we metabolise food. Weight gain during the menopause isn't inevitable though. You need to make a few small changes to your diet and exercise routine to maintain or improve your current weight and physique.

The menopause is a transition to the next stage of your life and you may feel it's time to make some changes. You need to create time and space for yourself to meditate and relax, develop your own interests and relationships, set new goals and to focus on your spiritual needs. Life coaching is a powerful method that helps you to work out what you want to do next and how to get there.

Sex and the Menopause (8)

Myths about sex and the menopause

- Sex is painful after the menopause.
- You lose interest in sex.
- Orgasms aren't the same anymore.
- Good sex has to be spontaneous.

Studies have shown that female sexual response (the ability to orgasm and desire for sexual touch) remain high as you get older and that many women remain sexually active into their 70s and beyond. The only thing that may change is vaginal dryness and lack of lubrication which can make sex, and the prospect of it, unappealing. This is linked to low levels of oestrogen in your body and can be remedied in several ways. Kathryn Colas, founder of Simply Hormones, recommends bio-identical hormones: 'I am using a bio-identical hormone compound of oestrogen and testosterone (very small dose) applied locally to the vagina – it's magic!' You can also use vaginal lubricants such as Yes or Replens. High quality fish oil supplements will also improve circulation in the genital area and throughout the body.

The sensual woman

It's a case of 'use it or lose it'. The more sex (and masturbation) you have, the more you want and the more your body comes to expect. You can take the time to discover what really turns you (and your partner) on and perhaps explore spiritual ideas about sex such as Tantra and Kabbalah. Monica Troughton, author, journalist and mentor to the Kabbalah Woman's Group, London, explains that Kabbalah is a belief system that can help you get more out of your life and relationships. 'I started my menopause and, instead of feeling ill, it made me feel womanly and sexy. My skin felt softer and my appetite changed. I had been vegetarian for 20 years but now felt the urge to eat meat. I listened to my body and had much more energy. Then I discovered Kabbalah,' she told Psychologies magazine (April 2009, 'Sex: How Other Women Do It'). This was the start of a spiritual journey for her that explored different ideas of sexuality and femininity. 'Sex was no longer a case of how to or how many but became charged with discovery and energy. It was wonderful to be fully present through sex', she explains.

After the menopause you don't have to worry about periods and contraception anymore. Older women come into their power sexually and younger men can be very attracted to the confidence and allure of women in their prime.

This is a good time to review your sexual script, make a few changes and try new things. It is very easy to get stuck in a rut with sex in a long term relationship, so the best form of foreplay initially is to talk about things. Your partner will be going through his own changes too and may be finding certain things difficult or challenging.

During the menopause certain physical changes are occurring which can (if not talked about and treated) lead to problems with sex. If your GP doesn't bring the subject up during your appointment, make sure you do.

How the menopause can affect sexual response

Common menopausal symptoms will have a knock-on effect on your sex life. It's hard to feel sensual and desirable when you're having hot flushes, sleeping badly and feeling preoccupied, anxious and stressed. If you're taking HRT and have gained a little weight, this may have an impact on your self-esteem too.

- Reduced levels of oestrogen and progesterone will have an impact on your sex drive and physical response. The vagina has lots of oestrogen receptors and the hormone helps to keep it moist, well lubricated, cleansed and responsive to touch. Lack of oestrogen means that the vagina and vulva become drier, shorter and the tissues are thinner due to loss of fat. Lubrication is slower and takes longer.
- The clitoris is covered by a tiny hood which protects it. When the tissues become thinner the hood can retract, leaving the clitoris exposed and too sensitive to touch. If you've previously enjoyed oral sex or direct clitoral stimulation, you may need to adapt techniques.
- As women's health writer Catherine Kalamis points out in her book Women Without Sex, during the menopause your sense of smell and touch can change which may influence how you respond physically to your partner. Our body's chemicals (pheromones) have a big part to play in attraction and if you can no longer smell your partner in the same way, it can affect levels of attraction and response.
- Certain medications and cancer treatments can cause vaginal dryness (chemotherapy and radiotherapy). Hysterectomy can also reduce blood flow, so more foreplay is necessary.
- If your skin becomes over-sensitive, hot flushes and night sweats may be intolerable. If there is stress in the bedroom over the room temperature, it is hardly likely that anything will lead to good sex. You may have noticed changes in skin sensitivity and how it feels to touch which will also affect your sexual response. Some women report a sensation of ants crawling on the skin, a process called formication, which is quite common.
- Lower levels of oestrogen can also affect how much saliva you produce which can have an impact on kissing and oral sex.

- Lower oestrogen levels mean less protection in the urinary tract, so you may experience more urinary and vaginal infections. In women the urinary tract is located close to the anus so cross-infection is easy if you wipe back to front, for example. Cystitis and thrush are two common infections that can impact on your sex life.
- A change in body shape and breast size and appearance may lead to you feeling less body confident. Skin also begins to sag as we get older due to loss of collagen and oestrogen.
- Orgasmic response can feel less intense due to nerve changes. However, it's not all bad news as www.netdoctor.co.uk's Dr David Delvin points out. Some women will be more orgasmic and multi-orgasmic after the menopause because they are less worried about getting pregnant, more relaxed about sex and more skilled at lovemaking. Mantak Chia's book The Multi-Orgasmic Woman explores this in detail. Sex therapist and Durex consultant Val Sampson suggests the following tip to improve your orgasms: breathe deeply and relax your tummy muscles as you approach climax for a more powerful, longer-lasting orgasm.
- Your ovaries continue to produce testosterone after they stop producing oestrogen and progesterone which can lead to a surge in libido at certain times of the month. Many women report feeling very sexually charged during the menopause.

Owning your sexuality

Evie Abston, a blogger at Good Vibrations sex store, runs workshops for menopausal women. She states that if you want to own your sexuality during and after the menopause, you need to approach this period in your life as a new sexual chapter. You need to be sexually adventurous as the same old tricks you've always used might not work anymore. Solutions to this, suggests sex educator Yvonne K Fulbright, include spending more time on foreplay, masturbating regularly, doing your pelvic exercises and experimenting with positions.

Talk about what is happening and new things you'd like to try. Evie points out that sexual arousal is mental as well as physical. It comes from what you are thinking about and focusing on during the day, so be mindful of this. Make sure you take time out to relax and be present in your body.

Evie suggests that this is a time to focus on yourself, your needs and what makes your heart sing. Make some physical changes to your appearance and take up new interests to stoke your passions. 'You can become a sexy dominant diva and ask your partner to feed you strawberries dipped in Belgian chocolate and give you a sensuous massage with an aromatic Jimmy Jane Bourbon massage candle. Have him massage every pleasure zone of your body', she states in her blog. 'The menopause doesn't mean the end of your sex life – just the end of your menstrual cycle and the claiming of your sexual rebirth. You should embrace the change and reinvent yourself,' she suggests.

Planning ahead

Sex is always part of a relationship, says Val Sampson. How good it is depends on the level of intimacy in your relationship. Are you leading disconnected lives? If so, try to build in fun and togetherness in your routine as a couple. Don't expect to have great sex if the intimacy isn't there. How intimate are you with friends and family? Are you open and affectionate? How do you respond to touch?

Communication and laughter are great aphrodisiacs. On a practical level, lubricant is a must. Some men regard using it as a failure, but it's a fact that all sexual activity is improved by using lubricant. Use a good quality, organic one that is bio-adhesive to moisturise the vaginal walls. This will make sex feel more pleasurable. Don't use massage oil as this blocks your vagina's ability to clean itself. Durex has a wide range of lubricants that you can find in the supermarket.

Don't get caught up in the myth that sex has to be spontaneous. Yes, spur of the moment fast sex is fun, but so is a slow, sensual planned encounter where you can both really devote time to pleasuring each other. There is research to show that once a woman begins to have sex she feels turned on. So, it's important not to wait for sexual desire to strike. Plan and schedule it. It can be fun to set aside some time. Use the build-up time to flirt and have fun. This will trigger your sex chemicals and put you in the mood.

Your brain is the biggest erogenous zone and female eroticism starts in the mind. To tap into this you need to consciously think about sex three or four times a day. Put a note in your diary to remind yourself. If you're working from home, take a break to masturbate and free up some energy and tension. Read some erotica and wear sensual fabrics to make you aware of your body and how it feels. Spend time thinking about sex and yourself as a sexual being. It is very easy to close your eyes and not notice male attention. 'I cheer now when I get a wolf whistle!' says life coach Carol Anne Rice.

Don't get hung up on penetrative sex as it can become a pressure. Research shows that this becomes less important as other forms of intimacy take over. Cooking together, sharing a bath, massage, watching a comedy and talking over a glass of good wine are all very powerful ways to feel connected. A woman's skin is 10 times more sensitive than a man's, so sensual touch can be more powerful and pleasurable than penetrative sex.

Experiment with positions

Experiment with positions, methods and speed of thrusting. You may find that slow and steady penetration to start with feels better. You can build up to a faster, deeper thrust once you are warmed up. Woman on top positions put you in control of depth and speed of penetration. Explore new scenarios to stimulate your mind – have sex outdoors and at different times of the day.

As we get older, we become less hung up on our looks and less inhibited. We become more comfortable with ourselves and our relationships. The level of intimacy, trust and connection is much greater, as is our knowledge of our partner, so it's worth building on this. Work out what areas need to be improved and talk about how you can do so.

Pelvic floor exercises

You can do all the exercise in the world, but if your pelvic floor isn't in good shape, you can kiss goodbye to a satisfying sex life. Experts talk about how a toned pelvic floor can help stress incontinence, but they don't talk about the more important things – it can give you stellar orgasms! A strong pelvic floor enables you to grip your partner while he is inside you, stimulate him to orgasm and experience full body orgasms yourself. What more incentive do you need?

How to do Kegels

Think of your pelvic floor muscles as a sling, lying along your pelvis. Its role is to hold things in place. However, the muscles are stretched and damaged during childbirth, so it's important to exercise them regularly.

To identify them, hold the flow of urine when you are on the toilet. Now, sit in a chair or lie on the floor and consciously squeeze them, quickly to begin with, hold for a second and release. Imagine you are travelling upwards in a lift and keep your back straight. Do 10-15 sets of fast squeezes and then slow it down. Squeeze for five seconds and hold for five seconds, not forgetting to breathe. Do these at least three times a week and you will notice a big difference within three months or so.

If you do yoga, speak to your yoga teacher and ask for a few moves. It's helpful to know how to do Kegel exercises in different positions – on your back and on all fours – to give them a deep workout. This is more challenging as it can be hard to find your pelvic floor muscles when on all fours, but it's worth persevering!

You can also buy machines to help you along such as weighted vaginal cones from Aquaflex. Copies of Kari Bø's Pelvicore DVD (www.corewellness.co.uk) are available free online (Kari Bø is an exercise scientist and core muscle expert).

The orgasmic diet

In her book, The Orgasmic Diet, Marrena Lindberg talks about how you can adapt your diet to increase your energy and libido. It's not a diet as such – you can still eat dark chocolate – but it involves supplementing your diet with high quality fish oils and multivitamins, eating balanced meals (higher in protein than carbohydrates) and cutting down on caffeine and sugars which stress the body and can impact on libido.

Marrena also recommends doing your Kegel exercises three times a week for a greater orgasmic response. It's a very inspiring read and well worth trying her recommendations for a few months to see the difference in how you feel. The starting point is taking an evening out (alone) to pamper yourself: have a warm bath and add sensual oils such as jasmine, ylang ylang or rose. The aim is to deeply relax and go to bed with yourself to figure out what you really like and what turns you on. Sounds obvious, but how many of us take the time and effort to do this for ourselves? Now is that time.

Talking about sex with your partner

'Keep things light when talking about sex', says Val Sampson. Remember the acronym BARE every time you want to discuss something sexual: B – breathe, A – accept what they have to say, R – respect them and don't say things you wouldn't want to hear yourself and E – eulogise, praise and say positive things. Use 'I' and 'we' rather than 'you' and 'your' to stay connected. Never talk about sex while you are in bed as you are both physically and psychologically vulnerable. It's better to talk about any issues or changes you'd like to make during a long walk.

Contraception and STIs

Experts recommend using contraception for a year after the age of 50 once your periods have stopped and two years prior to 50 to be safe from pregnancy. Your periods may be erratic but nature does have a sense of humour and there is a (remote) chance you may get pregnant. There has also been a rise in STIs in the over 50 age group. So, if you are enjoying sex with new partners, keep the condoms handy. Consult your local GUM clinic (genito-urinary clinic) for STI testing. You can find your nearest one via the Family Planning website: www.fpa.org.uk.

Checklist

- Organise an evening to yourself to devote to self-pleasure. Stock up on sensual oils, sex toys, lubricant and erotica. The goal is to really relax, explore your body and find out what really turns you on.
- Read Marrena Lindberg's book The Orgasmic Diet for inspiration.
- Work out a treatment plan for vaginal dryness if this is an issue.
- Think about ways you can relax and cut out stress from your life.
- Plan some sensual activities in the diary.
- Sign up for the free Pelvicore DVD and pencil in some regular time to do the exercises.

Summing Up

Female sexual response remains high as we get older and many women remain sexually active into their 70s and beyond. Common menopausal symptoms that affect your enjoyment of sex are vaginal dryness and lack of lubrication. Lack of oestrogen means the vagina and vulva become drier, shorter and the tissues thin due to loss of fat. Lubrication is slower and can take longer.

Vaginal dryness and lack of lubrication can be easily remedied via creams and hormones applied locally to the vagina. Talk to your partner and GP about any changes that are affecting your sexual response. You may find it embarrassing but rest assured, your GP has heard it all before!

Your ovaries continue to produce testosterone after they stop producing oestrogen and progesterone which can lead to a surge in libido at certain times of the month. Many women report feeling sexually charged during the menopause.

Approach this period in your life as a new sexual chapter. Spend more time on foreplay, masturbation and pelvic exercises and experiment with toys, locations and positions. If sex is important to you, it's vital to maintain regular sexual touch via intercourse or masturbation. Pelvic floor exercises can vastly improve orgasms and sexual response and you need to do them for at least three months initially to feel a difference.

Your Future Health (9)

This chapter is an overview of health conditions that could affect women in later life. It's for information only, so don't panic!

Hopefully, once you have reached the menopause and had your final period, many of the common symptoms described earlier will have diminished. Your hormone levels will have readjusted to new, lower levels or you may be supplementing them via HRT.

Oestrogen has a protective effect on the body, so as levels decrease it's important to review your health regularly and maintain a balanced lifestyle. As well as looking after your body, is also vital to keep your brain healthy with good support networks and interesting, challenging work and hobbies.

Keep a diary, noting any changes or symptoms you'd like to have checked. It's important to be aware of the most common health problems in older age, what causes them and what you can do now to prevent them. You will normally be offered regular medical screening for various conditions via the NHS or you can opt for private screening methods if you'd like a quicker result. Common health checks post-50 include mammography (breast check), a cervical smear test, eye tests, blood tests for high cholesterol and blood sugars, urine testing, pelvic examinations and a bone density scan to detect osteoporosis. It is also helpful to learn how to do breast self-examination. A Menocheck at the Marie Stopes Clinic will pick up any early problems and costs around £165. Ask your GP for further information.

The following health issues need to be monitored postmenopause.

Cardiovascular diseases (heart and circulatory)

Common cardiovascular diseases include atherosclerosis (hardening of the arteries), angina (chest pain caused by lack of blood circulation to the heart), heart attacks and strokes. Women are more at risk of these than various forms of cancer, yet we read far less about heart disease and women in the press.

Oestrogen has a protective effect on our heart, so prior to the menopause we are less at risk of developing problems. However, poor lifestyle habits become more of an issue postmenopause. You need to have regular medical checks to see if your cholesterol levels, blood sugar and blood pressure are within a normal range. High blood pressure is a major factor in cardiovascular diseases.

Heart disease is generally more serious for women because it is picked up later, and the obvious signs that men experience when having a heart attack aren't the same for women. Symptoms of a heart attack include nausea, breathlessness, dizziness, pain between the breasts and pain in the upper arms.

To maintain a healthy heart, you need to have the regular medical checks just mentioned. Make some lifestyle changes too – stop smoking, reduce stress, maintain a healthy, low (good) fat diet, monitor your alcohol intake and have a proper exercise and sleep routine. Studies have shown that taking a small dose (50mg) of aspirin a day can help prevent heart disease because it acts as a thinning agent – talk to your GP for advice.

Diabetes

Diabetes is when your body doesn't produce enough insulin and so is unable to metabolise sugar. As a result, sugar builds up in the bloodstream and leads to weight gain and long term health issues such as cardiovascular disease. It can also bring on a premature menopause. The most common type in older age is Type 2. Storing weight around your middle has been linked to insulin resistance, so you will need to keep a close eye on your weight and maintain a healthy lifestyle. For more information on diabetes, see Diabetes – The Essential Guide (Need2Know).

Osteoporosis

Bone is a living tissue and it changes throughout our life; old bone is replaced by new bone. We have our optimum bone strength around the age of 30, so it's important to try and build this up by eating a high calcium diet, having enough vitamin D (sunlight) and doing weight-bearing exercise such as walking or jogging. With osteoporosis, the bones have weakened to such a degree that fractures (mainly of the spine or hip in women) are common. This is hard to detect because there are no obvious physical signs until a fracture occurs, although you may notice a gradual loss of height as you get older.

Hip fracture is a serious issue because it can lead to loss of mobility and independent living. You are more at risk of osteoporosis if you have a poor diet, don't do regular weight-bearing exercise and have a premature menopause. Your GP or Well Woman Clinic will do a bone mineral density test to check how strong your bones are and note any weak areas. See www.nos.org.uk for further information.

Cancers

As we get older, the risk of certain cancers becomes greater. Studies have shown that there is a slight increased risk of breast cancer when a woman takes combined HRT for over five years, but see your GP for advice and guidance.

Breast cancer

Breast cancer is the most frequently diagnosed cancer in women. It is quite common for women to have fibrocystic changes during the perimenopause as hormone levels are unsettled. However, they will normally adjust after the menopause takes place. The best policy is to do a regular self-examination of your breasts at different times of your menstrual cycle if you are still having periods to familiarise yourself with your natural cyclic changes. For example, breasts tend to be lumpy and tender prior to your period, so it is especially important to check them after your period when hormone levels are lower. This will allow you to notice any unusual changes. If you are no longer menstruating, the timing is not as relevant.

If you are worried about a lump or discharge, speak to your GP or Well Woman Clinic. In most cases they will be benign. If a tumour does develop and is caught in the early stages (in the breast only), the prognosis is excellent. It is also reassuring to know that once you reach 50, you will be offered mammography every couple of years as a preventative measure. It's best to have this done after your period – when hormone levels are lower the breast tissue is less dense and easier to read.

Breast cancer has been linked to various factors – hereditary, a late menopause, childbearing after the age of 30 years, being overweight, lack of exercise and having a poor diet. For further information see Breakthrough Breast Cancer. Contact details can be found in the help list.

Uterine cancer (endometrial)

Statistics from www.menopause.org show that less than three out of 100 women over the age of 50 will develop uterine cancer, where cancerous cells start to develop on the endometrium (womb lining). Causes aren't specific but it has been linked to long-term exposure to oestrogen without the balance of progesterone (for example oestrogen-only HRT) which overstimulates the lining of the womb. Long-term use of the breast cancer drug Tamoxifen has also been linked to it but the risk here is very small.

Risk factors include late menopause (post 52), starting your periods early, obesity, diabetes and not having had children (your body has been exposed to oestrogen for longer).

Symptoms include unusual bleeding or discharge during perimenopause and low pelvic pain. You should always have any irregular or heavy bleeding checked out by a medical professional.

Cervical smear testing won't pick up any signs of uterine cancer, so annual pelvic examinations are recommended. Ultrasound testing will pick up any abnormalities. See your GP for further information.

Ovarian cancer

Ovarian cancer is the fifth most common cancer in women, with around 6,800 diagnoses a year in the UK according to support charity www.ovarian.org.uk. However, only around 11% of cases are diagnosed early, according to www.menopause.org, which means usually it has reached advanced stages and can be harder to treat.

Symptoms include persistent bloating, stomach or pelvic pain and feeling full very quickly.

There is a new blood test called the OvPlex Ovarian Cancer Diagnostic Test to detect early stages of the condition before treatment becomes difficult. There is further information on the developer's website: www.ovplex.com.au. An annual pelvic examination is also recommended. Talk to your GP for further information.

In the initial HRT and health trials, no link was found between HRT and ovarian cancer. There is no specific link to menopause with ovarian cancer.

Cervical cancer

This is cancer that develops on the cervix (neck of the womb). It affects around 2,800 women every year in the UK. It is caused by certain strains of the human papilloma virus (HPV). There are various symptoms and risk factors: vaginal discharge, painful sex, vaginal bleeding postmenopause, smoking, sexual activity from an early age and long-term use of the contraceptive pill. Being run down and having a weak immune system makes it harder for your body to fight off the HPV. You will be invited for cervical smear tests every five years between the ages of 25 and 60. This will pick up any pre-cancerous cells before they develop. A preventative vaccine is now offered to teenage girls and research is ongoing as to whether this would be beneficial to older women.

Cervical cancer has not been linked to the use of HRT.

Skin cancer

There are two main types of skin cancer: basal cell carcinoma and squamous cell carcinoma. Collectively, these are classed as non-melanoma and affect around 65,000 people every year in the UK. Basal is less aggressive – it grows slowly on the base epidermal layer in the form of a lump. Squamous can spread and typically forms on exposed areas of the skin – scalp, face, arms and legs. Skin cancer is caused by excess sun exposure, radiotherapy, working with chemicals and a low immune system.

Check your moles regularly and tell your GP about any changes you would like investigating. Always use a sunscreen when you are outside, even on cloudy days.

Pelvic and urinary health

Urinary incontinence

There are various forms of urinary incontinence and it's a problem that affects most women throughout life. The pelvic floor muscles take a hammering during childbirth and need strengthening up regularly via Kegel exercises. Urinary incontinence is caused by nerve and muscle damage and infection.

- Stress incontinence is when you leak urine while laughing, exercising, coughing or sneezing.
- Overflow incontinence happens when you aren't emptying your bladder properly – make sure you sit back on the toilet seat and avoid squatting.
- Urge incontinence is when you suddenly have to go and can't stop the urge.

See your GP or local continence clinic in the first instance. Dr Sarah Jarvis has some useful tips for handling incontinence, as mentioned in chapter 8.

Sexual health

It's important to look after your sexual health throughout your life. Being postmenopausal doesn't make you immune to sexually transmitted infections (over-50s are actually a high risk group). Divorce, new partners, testing boundaries and no fear of pregnancy means it's a bit more relaxed and easier to take risks. No one is hassling you about who you are sleeping with either!

Common STIs include chlamydia, genital herpes, HPV, genital warts (a strain of HPV) and gonorrhoea. It's important to stay safe and use good quality lubricants and condoms with new partners until you've both been tested. Vaginal skin is thinner as we age and more prone to tearing and discomfort through dryness.

Looking ahead

The perimenopause can be a stressful time, mostly because it's so unpredictable and you don't know what to expect from one day to the next. It is, however, a rite of passage, a transition to the next stage in your life and it helps to view it positively. Be inspired by the female centenarians of Okinawa, Japan. They live long, fruitful lives because of good dietary habits (low fat, low GI, high in phytoestrogens and only eating until you are ¾ full). They also take regular exercise, avoid stress and have a spiritual nature. According to the Okinawa Centenarian Study, women there tend to go through a natural menopause without taking drugs and experience (or report) fewer incidences of hot flushes and other health concerns.

Go and see the real life Body Worlds exhibition (www.bodyworlds.com) by German Anatomist Gunther von Hagens. It is a wonderful insight into how the human body works from conception to death. It puts the menopause into context and will make you see what an amazing creature you really are.

Checklist

- Find out what health checks you are entitled to now you've reached the menopause. Contact your local Well Woman Clinic.
- Find out about your family history – is there anything you need to be aware of?
- Go and see the Body Worlds exhibition for an inspirational look at the human body.
- Make some dietary changes to protect yourself against cardiovascular disease.

Summing Up

It's important to think about and prepare for your long-term health. Try and maintain a balanced lifestyle by not smoking, eating well and exercising. Regular health checks are available via your local Well Woman Clinic and the staff there will be able to advise you on what tests are required. Recommended health checks for the over 50s include a mammography (breast check), cervical smear test, eye tests, blood tests for high cholesterol, pelvic examinations and bone density scans. Organisations such as Bupa, Nuffield Health and the Marie Stopes Clinic offer these privately.

Cardiovascular disease (atherosclerosis, angina, heart attacks and strokes) is something that women need to be aware of. Oestrogen has a protective effect on the heart and this changes postmenopause. You can keep this in check by maintaining a healthy (low fat) diet, stopping smoking, exercising regularly, reducing your salt intake and having regular medical checks to test your blood pressure and cholesterol levels.

Osteoporosis is also more prevalent in later life. We have our optimum bone strength around the age of 30, after which it gradually weakens. This can lead to hip fractures and breaks in old age. Try and maintain your bone density levels by eating a high calcium diet, getting plenty of sunlight and doing weight-bearing exercises like walking and jogging.

Look after your sexual health. The over-50s age group are high risk when it comes to STIs, partly due to a more relaxed attitude to sex and new partners. Use good quality lubricants and condoms with a new partner until you have both been tested for STIs.

Your Stories (10)

On symptoms

'Hot flushes? I'm from Yorkshire – we don't do hot flushes up here…'

'Hot flushes, occasional night sweats and difficulty with concentration from time to time, accompanied by a general sense of not being on top of things intellectually. Sex is different but not painful due to a considerate partner. My mother's death (10 years ago) must have borne upon my symptoms. It precipitated me into an immediate cessation of menstruation.'

'I had some heavy periods at the beginning, lasting three weeks or more. The worst symptoms for me are hot flushes and night sweats which have plagued me for about five years now. I also notice that my facial skin is much drier.'

'I have been stressed about my family and my home for many years. My mother was ill for six years before her death two years ago and my daughter has ongoing personal and health problems. This has all been during the menopause so it is hard to say whether is has affected my symptoms at all. My instinct is that it hasn't affected them and that this is just how the menopause is.'

'The usual anxieties regarding teenagers and work in respect of the current climate – I don't believe these have any bearing on my symptoms.'

'For one day only I remember being aware that I was thinking like a different person to the one I was the day before.'

'I had weird hormone activity and sometimes felt very sexual in a way I don't recall being ever, but other times not at all. I had a tendency to slip off and sleep in a separate room to my husband as his snoring woke me (which obviously wasn't a problem throughout the rest of our marriage).'

'I am convinced that my teenagers and my workload had a negative bearing on my symptoms.'

'Heavy periods then lighter periods with extreme flooding which was totally unpredictable. I had my last period in January but then I immediately started getting hot flushes and night sweats.'

On lifestyle changes

'I'm reasonably healthy, a non-smoker and eat plenty of fruit, veg and fish. I'm told I look much younger than I am but I think this is down to genes (so did my mum!). I drink wine but no beer and hardly any spirits. I walk a lot as we live in the country and do lots of gardening. I put on too much weight when I hit the menopause but have lost quite a lot over the past year. I feel reasonably comfortable with myself somewhere between a size 14 and 16 (and I'm quite tall). I did this by listening to my own body and ignoring all of the advice to eat a big breakfast which has never suited me. I have a milky drink in the morning, a very light lunch and my main meal between 5pm and 6pm. I lost weight, felt fitter and stopped getting indigestion which had plagued me since the menopause. I have lost a bit more recently because my husband has had to change his diet for health reasons. I cut out red meat with him – it was never my favourite thing anyway.'

'My lifestyle is healthy. I'm a vegetarian and eat well. I probably look a little younger than I am. I'm aware that the skin dulls a bit but I think appearance is more about one's soul than about the hormones. My fitness is pretty good – I walk a lot. I accept it can't be like it was in my fell-running, cricket playing days! I haven't made any dramatic changes – I'm just listening to my body and acting accordingly.'

'I wonder if it might be worth looking at people's spiritual view in relation to life changes? I am a Quaker and have always believed that all stages of life are to be valued equally.'

‘My general lifestyle is healthy, as is my diet which has plenty of fruit and veg. I am fit and run regularly, including 5k and 10k races. I haven’t made any changes because of the menopause but I think that exercise helps me cope with it much better.’

‘I was at my peak in my 40s, was very busy, slim, had a good diet but always drank a bit too much. By my mid-50s I had gone off sex and was looking forward to a steady comfortable decline into old age (quite happily). Still doing yoga and walking daily with my dogs. Salt and pepper hair getting thinner, still very busy but tending to cut things out of my life I don’t want to do.’

‘I was reasonably fit – I swam two to three times a week. I thought my diet was good. I didn’t like my appearance and couldn’t control my weight gain. I changed my diet and exercise regime to include weight-bearing exercise, lost weight and changed the shape of my body.’

‘I was shown how to deal with my baggage and most issues are now resolved or “in progress”. I changed my lifestyle and working habits. My symptoms are no longer present (they can drag on until the end of a woman’s life).’

On HRT

‘My children left home and my marriage fell apart. I was diagnosed with osteoporosis at 55, almost by chance; my soon-to-be-ex-husband gave me a bear hug, not violently, just a big squeeze, and some ribs cracked. I went onto HRT which I’d previously been very sniffy about, and also Actonel (similar to Fosamax) on the advice of the Osteoporosis Society (not my GP or chiropractor, both of whom I suspect couldn’t properly understand the T and Z scores).

‘I loved HRT – it was like cycling backwards at speed. My hair got thicker again, I had much more energy and started looking for a lover. I came off it nearly two years ago. I still feel more active and physical, care what I look like and want to be part of things, more so than I did in my mid-50s (I’m nearly 61), but I’m happy to be at the age and condition I am. So far. I came off the Actonel after my third Dexa scan showed I was almost free of osteoporosis. I now have high blood pressure controlled by tablets. I’m active and happy.’

‘I sought advice on the menopause from a helpful female GP in our practice. She was very good – gave me the facts and figures and was supportive without browbeating me into anything. I tried HRT for about six months when my symptoms were at their worst and found that for half the month I was fine, but as soon as I added in the other hormone (progestogen) I was practically suicidal. My breasts, never small anyway, swelled up to pregnancy size and felt awful. I thought this couldn’t possibly be doing me any good. I just stopped taking the tablets. There were no ill effects. My chest went back to normal and I stopped being miserable. I would say that, in a way, it got me over a hurdle because, other than hot flushes, the worst of the symptoms never returned. I just didn’t like the way it made me feel, but then the pill has never agreed with me either.’

‘Unless menopausal symptoms are really debilitating, I think it unwise. Menopause is as natural as menarche. And who wants to be having periods when they’re 60?’

‘When I first went to a doctor about prolonged periods, he put me on HRT. It did control the bleeding but it made my legs very uncomfortable. I stopped taking it after three weeks. I wouldn’t take it again under any circumstances.’

‘Pretty scared, so trying to avoid it.’

‘Initially absolutely against it but loved it immediately when I started taking it. I used it for four to four and a half years and had to be almost forcefully taken off it. My osteoporosis has almost gone, my hair and skin are rejuvenated and I have more energy.’

‘In 1995 HRT was the new wonder drug – promoting longevity, preventing osteoporosis and relieving all menopausal symptoms. I went on it and as long as I didn’t complain, I wasn’t contacted after the Million Women Study was published. However, I discovered bio-identical hormone treatment and embarked on this course. It was very successful without the worry of exacerbating any potential breast cancer. I started the website www.simplyhormones.com as a result of being unable to find anyone that could “join up the dots”, talk to me in a holistic way that was reassuring and would allow me to make my own decisions.’

‘I think there should be a choice. When you’re climbing the walls you are looking for a magic pill to help quieten down those symptoms. HRT does not cause breast cancer but it can stimulate any cells if they are present. The risk is relative. Some cancer drugs cause heart problems but weighing up the risks, women go for the cancer drugs.’

‘I used HRT for about three years and I had a Mirena coil fitted (slow release progestogen). I had the coil removed as my consultant agreed it wasn’t doing much for me. It did resolve the hot flushes, sweating and joint pain but not much else. I was mildly depressed and didn’t realise it so other treatments were later recommended (cognitive behavioural therapy).’

On supplements and complementary therapies

‘I used black cohosh to help with hot flushes which people now say is dangerous (it has been linked to liver damage), but it was excellent for me (and I didn’t take it for too long). I also took sage and various other supplements. The thing that helped the hot flushes most was three sessions of acupuncture – it was miraculous. They just faded and went within the space of a couple of weeks and have never really come back.’

‘Black cohosh helped with flushes and night sweats.’

‘My menopause symptoms started two years ago when I was 46. The main problem was hot flushes and night sweats which stopped me sleeping properly. I went for nine months without a proper night’s sleep. I went to see my GP who was reluctant to put me on HRT as I had previously had a deep vein thrombosis (DVT). The problem was he didn’t really come up with any alternatives for me either.

‘Eventually I went back to him and said I didn’t care about the associated risks, I just needed something to help me. This time I saw a locum who put me on betablockers to lower my heart rate. They helped for a short while but then the flushes returned and I felt no further forward.

‘A patient (at work) told me about VitalWOMAN and how the tablets had helped her daughter-in-law. They have been a lifesaver. I no longer experience hot flushes and night sweats which means I sleep better and am not so irritable and moody – better for me, my family and work colleagues.’

‘I take Kalms regularly but think they only sometimes work.’

‘I have just ordered Peruvian Maca and was going to try black cohosh but, in view of recent publicity with respect to liver damage, have decided against it.’

‘Tried mixtures of minerals and herbs designed for postmenopausal women for a bit as I was afraid I’d shrivel like a prune, but I did not notice the difference when I stopped taking them.’

On getting older

'I'm quite positive. I don't much like getting older but this has more to do with how other people perceive you I think. I'm a writer and there's a sense in which you have to stay looking reasonably young or people patronise. Somebody called me "dear" the other week. I have now primed myself so that the next person to do that will be called "darling" in return. I used to suffer from PMS so it's wonderful not to have periods anymore. I've also noticed that my creativity seems to have increased by leaps and bounds. It feels quite empowering. I just wish I had had this amount of confidence and wisdom when I was younger!'

'Sometimes I feel stressed about work – or about not making enough money. I've been a freelance my whole life which means that I've always lived precariously. Living like that when you grow older is a little daunting. On the other hand, there's a freedom to growing older that is unexpectedly exciting. I have a 22-year-old son and also work part-time with students. I like young people very much and find that I like to keep up with technology, etc. I think keeping interested and positive helps. I also have some very inspirational older friends.'

'I should be stressed financially and with the massive structural problems to the access of my house – but I'm not. I feel very lucky and look back upon my life as always having been so (never had much money, never will have). I think the post-war generation were exceedingly fortunate – free education, pre-HIV and Aids and Thatcher's selling-off of the housing stock etc.'

On the menopause

'I think it is positive. I have few regrets about growing older and I welcome the stability and confidence that comes with maturity. No further possibility of pregnancy has a liberating feel to it which makes for more relaxed lovemaking.'

‘I feel indifferent to it. I view it as a natural process and keep myself busy. I have never dwelt upon it or worried about it. I do think it’s a positive thing to be free of monthly periods.’

‘I have found it helpful to think about the menopause as little as possible and not to dwell upon symptoms or related issues. Sometimes it is good to talk to other women in similar positions – it makes you feel less alone and more normal. I have followed my instincts, not been influenced by any particular idea or therapies, foods or drinks and have just carried on as usual.’

‘I love it. I’d like to stay this age. I don’t have the urges to go out and be part of the scene but do have the energy to be fairly physical. However, I realise my restrictions (I gave up physical theatre). I have a full circle of friends, especially other artists. I don’t get anxious. I feel I am quite realistic and still optimistic – I almost feel sensible! I have lost a lot of my ambition – I don’t wish to be better than other people or to win. It’s very important to me to be working in creative ways with other people which I have always done.’

‘I think keeping a diary log would be beneficial.’

‘It was a negative time in my life to begin with but now I have found my own path to wellness again. I urge women to approach menopausal symptoms sooner rather than later – the sooner, the better – I believe a natural pathway can be successful but you must be committed to making changes to your lifestyle.’

‘Women are going through a metamorphosis and this psychological and physiological process should be a good experience; learning how to deal with the process should be made easier.’

‘Lack of information for men just seems to aggravate the problem – it’s like the blind leading the blind.’

‘The forums on www.allaboutyou.com are very good. I wish I had found them before then I would have realised it wasn’t only me. I’m not worried about it and feel that having no periods is a bonus.’

On sex

'Sexually, things are improving but very slowly. I've been with my husband since 1980, so I suspect it's only to be expected. We had a real dip when I was in the middle of all the menopausal symptoms but now things are slowly getting better. I suspect I'm as capable as anyone younger of falling madly in love and of responding physically, so I think any change in sexual response is to do with the familiarity of a long-term partner rather than the menopause – and possibly to be expected. Conversations with female friends would suggest that most of us experience something similar.'

'Response is slower. Libido is reduced though I'm still there! I'm not troubled by this.'

'I feel the same as I did, with what I would say was a normal libido and response, although perhaps tiredness affects that at times.'

'I've been with my partner for five years. Sex isn't part of our relationship now, although it was at first. This has got more to do with his antidepressants and lowered libido, but I'm happy with just the affectionate side of things.'

'I feel more like the person I was before puberty. As I'm now out of the habit of having regular sex, I would not wish to start again. I thought I'd feel sad, but I don't. I like being a non-sexual person, but I don't want to look like a frump.'

'I totally went off sex, mostly because (I now realise) I knew I had dried up and not only was it painful but I knew I wasn't going to reach orgasm. I am using a bio-identical hormone compound of oestrogen and testosterone (very small dose) applied locally – it's magic!'

On mothers

'She always taught me that it was just another stage of life and not something to dread or obsess about. Her menopause was prematurely precipitated by my father's death when she was 45.'

'I remember her complaining about hot flushes.'

'I recall my mother having polyps in her womb in the period leading up to her menopause. She was advised by the GP not to have a hysterectomy but to have something else, whereby the house smelled terrible for a while. Funnily enough, she doesn't remember! She had her menopause a bit later than me. It was shrouded by my father having a heart attack and eventually dying. She was helping my sister and her children a lot so we never really talked about it much. She is still alive at 91, living independently and with a better memory than mine! She never did like alcohol much...'

'I remember that she would turn down the central heating thermostat and I, a teenager, would turn it up! She did leave home for three days when I was about 19 saying she couldn't cope with things at home (blaming my father) and she had to get away. When she returned the subject was never broached in my company and I felt uneasy about asking her – she was very cold emotionally.'

On inspiring women

'My friend Scottish poet Sheila Templeton has written a superb poem (in Scots) about the menopause. It can be found at the link http://www.scottishcorpus.ac.uk/corpus/search/document.php?documentid=1490. Says it all, really!'

'A very amusing book called What A Woman of Forty-Five Ought To Know by Emma Frances Angell Drake, and Marilyn Glenville's book New, Natural Alternatives to HRT, which explores nutrition and menopause and views it as a natural process, not a disease, are both supportive and helpful.'

Summing Up

This chapter is a selection of viewpoints and personal experiences of the menopause from the women interviewed for this book. It does not represent the views of the author and aims to show how women's experiences can vary. Consult your GP if you would like further advice or clarification on any of the opinions, products and services stated here.

Help List

There are several organisations providing up-to-date information on the menopause, women's health, HRT and CAM. The Internet is a useful starting point for your research although the quality of health information varies. It's best to seek out websites with professional advisory boards, such as those listed below. It's also worth speaking to your GP and local menopause clinic about your options, as your GP will have your medical history and up-to-date information about treatment options.

Allied Aromatherapy Practitioners' Association (AAPA)

The AAPA, 14 Orleans Road, Upper Norwood, London SE15 3TA
Tel: 0208 653 9152
enquiries@aapa.org.uk
www.aapa.org.uk
A non-profit association dedicated to the development of aromatherapy and the support of therapists.

The Association of Reflexologists

5 Fore Street, Taunton, Somerset, TA1 1HX
Tel: 01823 351 010
info@aor.org.uk
www.aor.org.uk
The Association of Reflexologists (AoR) is a non-profit membership organisation providing support to professionally qualified practitioners. You can use the website to search an online database of practitioners in your area.

Ayurvedic Medical Association UK

59 Dulverton Road, Selsdon, South Croydon, Surrey, CR2 8PJ
Tel: 0208 657 6147
The Ayurvedic Medical Association UK is the professional body for the qualified Ayurvedic practitioners. There are about 25-30 qualified Ayurvedic physicians in the UK who are registered with the Ayurvedic Medical Association UK. They hold malpractice insurance

and maintain a code of ethics.

The Bach Centre

www.bachcentre.com
Visit the website for information on the different remedies available, advice and case studies.

Breakthrough Breast Cancer

246 High Holborn, London, WC1V 7EX
Tel: 0207 025 2400
info@breakthrough.org.uk
www.breakthrough.org.uk
Leading UK charity committed to fighting breast cancer through research, education and campaigning.

British Acupuncture Council

63 Jeddo Road, London, W12 9HQ
Tel: 0208 735 0400
info@acupuncture.org.uk
www.acupuncture.org.uk
The UK's main regulatory body for practice of traditional acupuncture by over 2,800 acupuncturists.

The British Complementary Medicine Association

PO Box 5122, Bournemouth, BH8 0WG
Tel: 0845 345 5977
office@bcma.co.uk
www.bcma.co.uk
Information about complementary therapies, including a therapist finder service.

British Holistic Medical Association

5 Sea Lane Close, East Preston, West Sussex BN16 1NQ
www.bhma.org
Support and advice for people wishing to find out about holistic treatments and preventative measures. Produces the Journal of Holistic Healthcare.

The British Menopause Society

4-6 Eton Place, Marlow, Buckinghamshire, SL7 2QA
Tel: 01628 890 199
admin@thebms.org.uk
www.thebms.org.uk
A registered charity for UK health professionals and those working within reproductive health. Provides information about menopause, conferences, lectures, meetings and exhibitions.

The Daisy Network

PO Box 183, Rossendale, BB4 6WZ
daisy@daisynetwork.org.uk
www.daisynetwork.org.uk
Provides factsheets and information about premature menopause and the health issues surrounding it.

The Hysterectomy Association

West View, West Street, Broadwater, Dorchester, Dorset DT1 3QQ
info@hysterectomy-association.org.uk
www.hysterectomy-association.org.uk
Information to help women make the right choices about hysterectomy.

Menopause.org

5900 Landerbrook Drive, Suite 390, Mayfield Heights OH 44124 USA
info@menopause.org
www.menopause.org
Website of the North American Menopause Society, a non-profit scientific organisation that promotes women's health and understanding of the menopause. Accurate information about the menopause, perimenopause, early menopause, symptoms and long-term health issues. Includes strategies and therapies to enhance health, including HRT and bio-identical hormones.

The Menopause Exchange

PO Box 205, Bushey, Herts, WD23 1ZS

Tel: 0208 420 7245
info@menopause-exchange.co.uk
www.menopause-exchange.co.uk
An independent organisation providing up-to-date information on the menopause and related topics, including medical conditions, HRT, complementary therapies, nutrition and self-help. Produces a regular newsletter about the menopause.

Menopause Matters

info@menopausematters.co.uk
www.menopausematters.co.uk
An independent, clinician-led website providing current information about the menopause, symptoms, HRT and other treatment options. It aims to help women make a more informed choice about their menopause and how to manage it.

National Institute of Medical Herbalists

Clover House, James Court, South Street, Exeter EX1 1EE
Tel: 01392 426 022
info@nimh.org.uk
www.nimh.org.uk
The UK's leading professional body representing herbal practitioners.

National Osteoporosis Society

Camerton, Bath, BA2 0PJ
Tel: 01761 471 771
info@nos.org.uk
www.nos.org.uk
UK charity dedicated to improving diagnosis, prevention and treatment of osteoporosis. It has a helpline service for medical queries, information about osteoporosis and access to local support groups.

NHS Choices

Tel: 0845 4647 (NHS Direct)
www.nhs.uk

Comprehensive information service for everyday healthcare needs. Lifestyle advice and practical help finding and using NHS services in the UK. You can find medical advice, search for services in your area and compare hospitals.

Office of Dietary Supplements (National Institute of Health)

6100 Executive Blvd, Room 3B01, MSC 7517, Bethesda, MD 20892-7517
ods@nih.gov
http://ods.od.nih.gov/index.aspx
Factsheets about nutritional supplements.

The Okinawa Centenarian Study

www.okicent.org
The Okinawa Centenarian Study looks at genetic and lifestyle factors responsible for low illness rates, positive menopause and a long life expectancy in Okinawa, Japan.

Simply Hormones

PO Box 218, Uckfield, East Sussex, TN22 3YT
kathryn@simplyhormones.com
01825 700492
www.simplyhormones.com
Kathryn Colas organises Time of Your Life menopause roadshows and runs a subscription-based website providing information about the menopause, symptoms, HRT, hysterectomy, osteoporosis and complementary therapies.

Society of Homeopaths

11 Brookfield, Duncan Close, Moulton Park, Northampton, NN3 6WL
Tel: 0845 450 6611
info@homeopathy-soh.org
www.homeopathy-soh.org
The largest organisation registering professional homeopaths in Europe.

Society of Teachers of the Alexander Technique

1st Floor, Linton House, 39-51 Highgate Road, London, NW5 1RS
Tel: 0207 482 5135
office@stat.org.uk
www.stat.org.uk
The oldest and largest professional society of teachers of the Alexander technique.

Wallace-Kelsey Foundation

www.wallacekelsey.org.uk
Official website for the Wallace-Kelsey test.

Women's Health Concern (WHC)

4-6 Eton Place, Marlow, Bucks, SL7 2QA
Tel: 01628 478 473
pshervington@womens-health-concern.org
www.womens-health-concern.org
An independent service providing information about the menopause and women's health issues. Telephone and email counselling support available from nurses and medical advisers.

WPF Therapy

23 Magdalen Street, London, SE1 2EN
Tel: 0207 378 2000
reception@wpf.org.uk
www.wpf.org.uk
A leading charitable provider of therapy in the UK, established since 1969. Provides high quality, affordable psychodynamic counselling, psychotherapy and group therapy.

Integrated health clinics

The Health Doctors

121 Harley Street, London W1G 6AX
Tel: 0207 224 2423
www.thehealthdoctors.co.uk

Medical clinic providing information about integrated medicine, bio-identical hormones, nutrition, osteopathy, western herbal medicine, homeopathy, NLP, massage, yoga and more.

The Holistic Medical Clinic

19 Wimpole Street, London, W1G 8GE
Tel: 0207 631 1111
info@holisticmedical.co.uk
www.holisticmedical.co.uk
Medical clinic providing information about bio-identical hormones, the male andropause, positive ageing, preventative medicine, sexual dysfunction, counselling, nutritional medicine, acupuncture, stress management and more.

Menopause products and resources

Chillow Pillow

Soothsoft Ltd, Unit 10, North Estate, Old Oxford Road, Piddington, High Wycombe, Buckinghamshire, HP14 3BE
Tel: 01494 88 2224
info@soothsoft.co.uk
www.chillow.co.uk
A 2cm thick personal cooling pad that reduces core body temperature to induce sleep naturally. It can be used on top of or inside your pillowcase.

Estroven

www.estroven.com
A natural product that provides nutritional support during the menopause. It contains natural isoflavones from soya, Japanese Arrowroot and essential vitamins and minerals.

LadyCare

Lady Care Lifetime Ltd, 24 Emery Road, Bristol, BS4 5PF
Tel: 0117 9710 710
www.ladycare-uk.com

A magnetic device that helps to balance mood and alleviate physical symptoms of menopause. It is worn over the pelvic area and is clipped to your underwear. Available from pharmacies or online via the website and costs £19.95.

Linda Kearns' Menopause Cake

Wellfoods Ltd, Unit 6, Mapplewell Business Park, Mapplewell, Barnsley, South Yorkshire, S75 6BS
Tel: 01226 381 712
www.wellfoods.co.uk
A 'HRT alternative' cake that contains nutrients to help women through the menopause. It contains soya milk, soya flour, pumpkin seeds, raisins, linseeds, sesame seeds, nuts and dried fruits.

Menopace

Vitabiotics Ltd, 1 Apsley Way, London, NW2 7HF
Tel: 0208 955 2600
www.menopace.com
A formulation of 21 nutrients which can be taken with or without HRT to provide nutritional support. Tablets include vitamins B and C, zinc, magnesium and soy isoflavones.

Pelvicore Pelvic Toning DVD

SCA Hygiene Products, Freepost TENA
Tel: 0845 30 80 803
www.corewellness.co.uk
A DVD programme to help support your health and wellbeing. Core muscle expert Kari Bø has produced the Pelvicore technique – simple exercises that will tone your pelvic muscles. You can order a free DVD via the website.

Replens long-lasting personal lubricant

www.replens.com
A long-lasting feminine moisturiser that can help relieve vaginal dryness. It delivers moisture for up to three days so you don't need

to apply it before sex. It helps to rejuvenate the vaginal lining, eliminate dry skin cells and replenish the vagina's natural moisture levels.

VitalWOMAN

Simply Vital Ltd, Houghton-le-Spring, Tyne & Wear, DH5 8QA
Tel: 0870 609 1180
www.simplyvital.com
A natural supplement containing phystoestrogens – plant oestrogens that can help redress low levels of oestrogen in the body and reduce menopausal symptoms.

Wild Mexican Yam

www.wildmexicanyam.co.uk
A history of the development of Wild Mexican Yam as an alternative to HRT.

Yes Organic Personal Lubricants

www.yesyesyes.org
Soil Association certified organic water and oil-based personal lubricant. It enhances sexual pleasure and helps to remoisturise vaginal tissues during the menopause.

Zestra Arousal Oil

Zestra (UK) Ltd, 23 Cranley Gardens, London, N10 3AA
Tel: 0845 658 8877
customer.services@zestra.com
www.zestra.co.uk
Topical product clinically proven to increase female sexual arousal, desire, sensation and sexual pleasure.

Magazines & blogs

Better Than I Ever Expected: Straight Talk About Sex After Sixty

www.betterthanieverexpected.blogspot.com

Joan Price's blog celebrates the joys and addresses the challenges of elder sexuality. Joan is the author of Better Than I Ever Expected: Straight Talk About Sex After Sixty. Her blog covers senior sex news and views, tips and reviews.

Feminine Zone

www.femininezone.com
Online magazine for women. Explores sex and sensuality in mid-life and other health and lifestyle issues.

Good Housekeeping

www.goodhousekeeping.com
Menopause and health forums on the website.

Psychologies

www.psychologies.co.uk
Magazine exploring self-knowledge, family, parenting, relationship, wellbeing and sexual issues.

Book List

Better Than I Ever Expected: Straight Talk About Sex After Sixty
By Joan Price, Avalon Publishing Group, New York, Reprint Edition, 2005.

Eat To Beat Menopause: Over 100 Recipes to Help You Overcome Symptoms Naturally
By Linda Kearns, Thorsons, UK, 2001.

Hot Flushes, Cold Science: A History of the Modern Menopause
By Louise Foxcroft, Granta Books, London, First Edition, 2009.

Is It Me Or Is It Hot In Here?: A Modern Woman's Guide To The Menopause
By Jenni Murray, Vermilion, London, 2003.

The Menopause – Ask The Experts
By Norma Goldman, Hammersmith Press Limited, London, 2009.

The Multi-Orgasmic Woman: Discover Your Full Desire, Pleasure, and Vitality
By Mantak Chia and Rachel Carlton Abrams, Rodale Press, Pennsylvania, 2006.

Natural Progesterone: Effective, Safe Treatment for Menopausal Symptoms, PMS and other Hormone-Related Problems
By John Lee, Ann Rushton and Shirley Bond, Thorsons, UK, 1999.

New Natural Alternatives to HRT
By Marilyn Glenville PhD, Kyle Cathie Ltd, London, 2003.

The Optimized Woman: Using Your Menstrual Cycle to Achieve Success and Fulfillment: If You Want to Get Ahead, Get a Cycle
By Miranda Gray, O Books, (Nationwide), 2009.

The Orgasmic Diet: Boost Your Libido and Achieve Orgasm
By Marrena Lindberg, Piatkus Books, London, 2007.

The Sexy Years: Discover the Hormone Connection: The Secret to Fabulous Sex, Great Health, and Vitality, for Women and Men
By Suzanne Somers, Three Rivers Press, London, 2005.

The Silent Passage: Menopause
By Gail Sheehy, Pocket Books, US, Revised Edition, 1998.

The Technology of Orgasm: Hysteria, the Vibrator and Women's Sexual Satisfaction
By Rachel P Maines, The John Hopkins University Press, Maryland, 2001.

Need - 2 - Know

Other Large Print Titles Include ...

Allergies A Parent's Guide
ISBN 978-1-86144-160-7 £12.99

Autism A Parent's Guide
ISBN 978-1-86144-165-2 £12.99

Drugs A Parent's Guide
ISBN 978-1-86144-136-2 £12.99

Dyslexia A Parent's Guide
ISBN 978-1-86144-138-6 £12.99

Bullying A Parent's Guide
ISBN 978-1-86144-137-9 £12.99

Epilepsy The Essential Guide
ISBN 978-1-86144-152-2 £12.99

Teenage Pregnancy The Essential Guide
ISBN 978-1-86144-139-3 £12.99

Gap Years The Essential Guide
ISBN 978-1-86144-169-0 £12.99

How to Pass Exams A Parent's Guide
ISBN 978-1-86144-140-9 £12.99

Child Obesity A Parent's Guide
ISBN 978-1-86144-141-6 £12.99

Applying for a Job The Essential Guide
ISBN 978-1-86144-180-5 £12.99

ADHD The Essential Guide
ISBN 978-1-86144-145-4 £12.99

Student Cookbook – Healthy Eating
The Essential Guide
ISBN 978-1-86144-146-1 £12.99

Stress The Essential Guide
ISBN 978-1-86144-147-8 £12.99

Your First Pregnancy The Essential Guide
ISBN 978-1-86144-158-4 £12.99

Special Educational Needs A Parent's Guide
ISBN 978-1-86144-149-2 £12.99

The Pill An Essential Guide
ISBN 978-1-86144-150-8 £12.99

University A Survival Guide
ISBN 978-1-86144-153-9 £12.99

Visit **www.need2knowbooks.co.uk** for the full range. To order our titles call **01733 898103**, email **sales@n2kbooks.com** or visit the website. Selected ebooks available online.

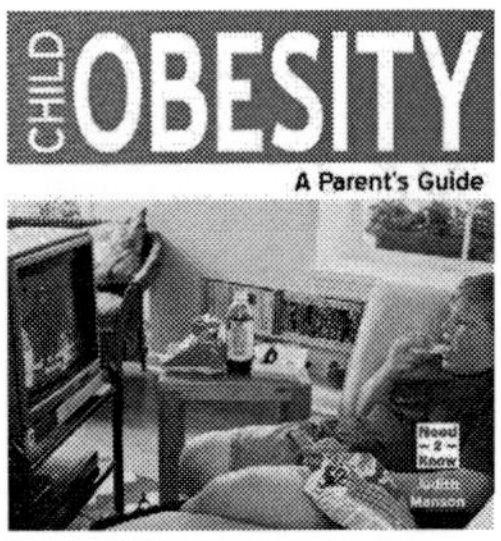

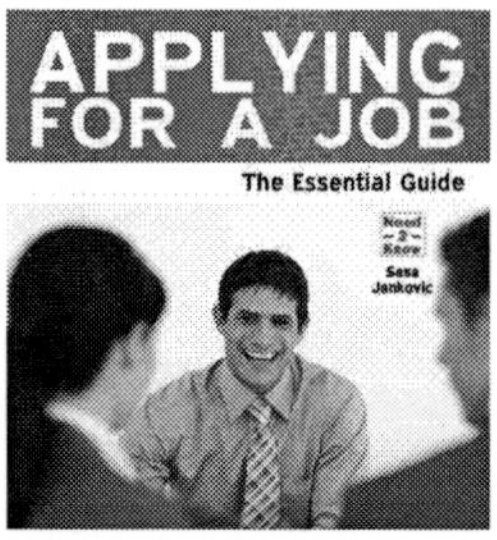

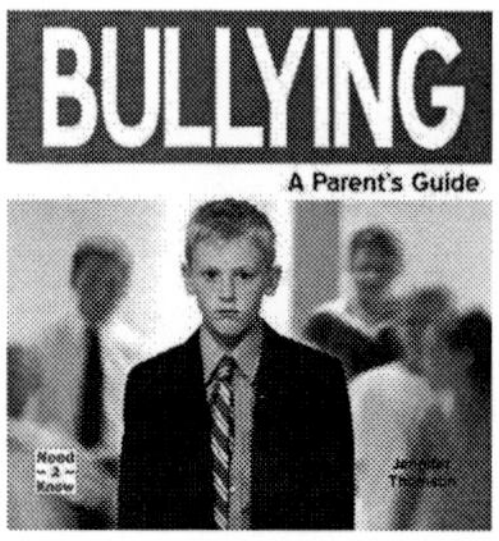

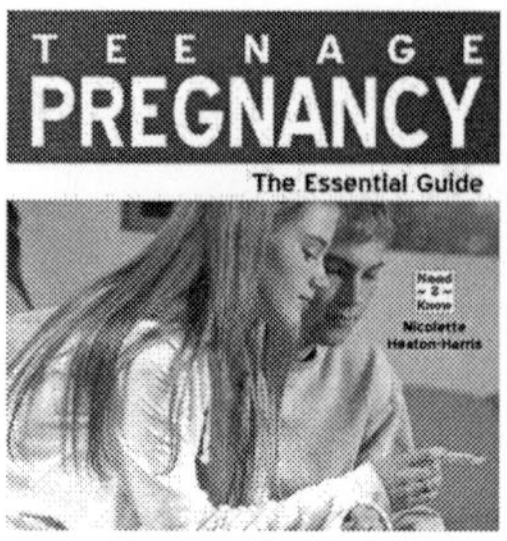

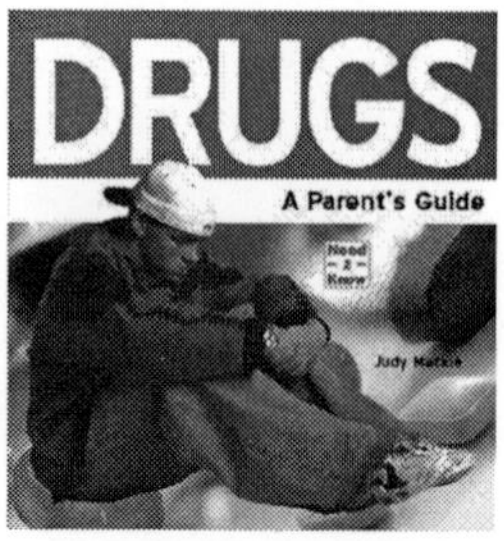

Need - 2 - Know, Remus House, Coltsfoot Drive, Peterborough, PE2 9BF